SPARKS OF DIVINITY

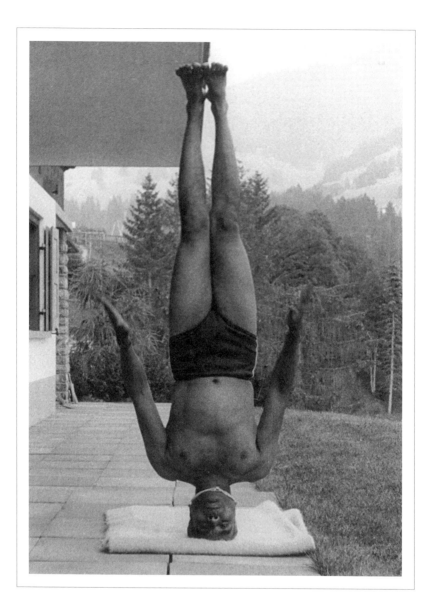

SPARKS OF DIVINITY

THE TEACHINGS OF

B.K.S. IYENGAR

FROM 1959 TO 1975

Compiled by
Noëlle Perez-Christiaens

RODMELL PRESS • BERKELEY, CALIFORNIA • 2012

Printed in the United States of America
ISBN 1-978-930485-32-7

Library of Congress Cataloging-in-Publication Data
is available.

Project Editor: Donald Moyer
Coeditor: Holland Hammond
Production Editor: Linda Cogozzo
Indexer: Ty Koontz
Cover and Text Design: Gopa & Ted2, Inc.
Cover Photograph: Steve Baczewski
Author Photograph: Danielle Garnier
Lithographer: Walsworth Print Group
Text set in Arno Pro
Distributed by Publishers Group West

Contents

Acknowledgments

WITH HEARTFELT THANKS to Noëlle Perez-Christiaens for compiling and preserving these wonderful teachings of B.K.S. Iyengar and for remaining steadfast in her conviction that Iyengar should be heard in his own voice and his own words, enigmatic though they may be. We are grateful to Noëlle for allowing Rodmell Press to publish this new edition.

With gratitude to B.K.S. Iyengar for providing the photographs reproduced in this book, and for the continued inspiration of his teachings. The passage of thirty-five years has not dimmed the brilliance of his insights.

With deep appreciation for the enormous contribution of Georgia and Philippe Leconte, who were entrusted by Noëlle with overseeing this revised edition of *Sparks of Divinity* on her behalf. Georgia and Philippe not only wrote the foreword and afterword but also selected excerpts from *B.K.S. Iyengar: Un Mystique Hindou Ivre de Dieu* for inclusion in this book.

Georgia and Philippe collaborated with Noëlle on the original French translation of *Sparks of Divinity*, and their skill in deciphering Iyengar's most cryptic sayings often gave me a clue on how to clarify the English text without diluting the impact of Iyengar's words. It has been a great pleasure to work with such dedicated, knowledgeable, and generous colleagues.

Many thanks to Jean Couch of the Balance Center in Palo Alto, CA, for arranging the historic meeting with Georgia and Philippe Leconte at Venus Restaurant, in Berkeley, and for reading and commenting on their introductory material. We are grateful to Thea Sawyer for her fine translation of the foreword, afterword, Noëlle's Indian Journal, and the Early Life of B.K.S. Iyengar.

Final thanks to our coeditor, Holly Hammond, for her insightful suggestions on how to organize the material in this book, and to Vicky Palmer for her perceptive reading of *B.K.S. Iyengar: Un Mystique Hindou Ivre de Dieu.*

Donald Moyer, Publisher
Rodmell Press

Foreword

SPARKS OF DIVINITY is a collection of sayings from yoga master B.K.S. Iyengar, compiled and edited by Noëlle Perez-Christiaens, one of his first Western students. Noëlle first published the book in 1976 in a French and English bilingual format. At that same time, she published a second book in French only, titled *B.K.S. Iyengar: Un Mystique Hindou Ivre de Dieu*. These two books complement each other. The first one quotes the master himself; the second one is filled with anecdotes and observations from Noëlle's encounters with this exceptional man who has inspired her all her life.

This new edition of *Sparks of Divinity* includes the English text from the first edition, plus extracts from *B.K.S. Iyengar: Un Mystique Hindou Ivre de Dieu*, including excerpts from the journal Noëlle kept during the time she studied one-to-one with Iyengar in India, and subsequent chapters that chronicle the early life of Iyengar, his work, and his family.

Who was this brave young woman who traveled alone to India in 1959? Noëlle Perez-Christiaens, then thirty-three years old, was forever the student. Her search was spiritual: religious studies at the Catholic Faculty in Paris, biblical studies, Catholic liturgy, and study of Eastern and Western mysticism. She searched passionately and persistently.

From an early age, she had been drawn to the great spiritual traditions of

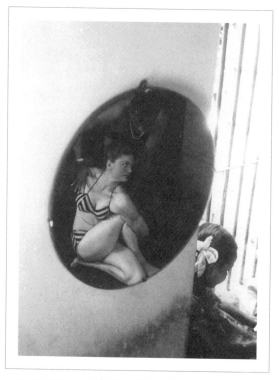

the East, inspired by reading *Voyage d'une Parisienne à Lhassa* (*My Journey to Lhasa*) by Alexandra David Neel. In search of contemplative techniques, she embarked upon yoga, and within two years had read all the literature available to her on the subject. Over the next four years, she studied with several teachers who practiced in France and Switzerland, and then taught her own yoga class. But India was calling.

An employee at the Indian Tourist Office introduced Noëlle to a former colonel who had worked with T. Krishnamacharya in Mysore as well as with his student, B.K.S. Iyengar, in Pune. He is the one who introduced her to Iyengar.

Noëlle cobbled together the money needed to pay for her trip, her stay, and the tuition. Her first class with Iyengar was on July 14, 1959. To her surprise, she found it "just a special gymnastics without any spirituality." However, she decided to stay, due to the "precise and refined technique" of the master.

Gradually she discovered that even if contemplation was not ostensibly part of the practice, what she found there was a confrontation with the self that could widen the will: the will for perfection in the pose, the will to become aware, and the will to develop concentration.

It was a turning point in her life. She had found her mentor and guide. A new path opened, and she did not stray from it. She never returned to India, but attended Iyengar's classes during several summers in Gstaad, Switzerland, where he was invited by Yehudi Menuhin. And Iyengar came to Paris in 1971, 1972, and 1976 to teach at the Institute B.K.S. Iyengar, which Noëlle founded after her return from Pune. She sent him countless students, one of them being Georgia, her "spiritual daughter" and one of her most enlightened students, who spent four months in Pune in 1974.

Sparks of Divinity

Noëlle's notebooks were full of the master's remarks about how to see the world, the philosophy of yoga, his devotion to the Divine, and his love of human beings. In 1974 she asked herself, Do I have the right to keep this great beacon of light for myself and my students, to clarify our path only? She wrote to Iyengar and made him part of her project to write a book "about everything except the technique of yoga."

On June 18, 1974, Iyengar answered: "In regard to the book you plan to write, I have no objection whatsoever; go ahead. And ask Beatrice Harthan in my name to send you 'the list' she has put together. Ask also Silva Mehta. You can write about this to Lyn Dorfling in Transvaal so she can send you what she wrote down. Someone else has taken many notes; it is Winnie Young from Natal. Kareen could also have something. All those collections can be added to your work."

Then, Noëlle says, "A fire was lit in me. I wrote in all directions."

By October 1974, she had nearly a thousand index cards, translated by friends and students so that each card would be bilingual. At Christmastime the manuscript was ready for photocopying so the whole thing could be taken to Iyengar by two students on their way to Pune for the inauguration of the new institute in January 1975. Three weeks later, everything came back in the suitcase of another student. Each card had been reviewed and corrected. Then each card was typed and translated again and linked to an index of sixty key words. Noëlle wrote: "Our treasure was ready to light the way for all who were trying to educate, refine, and purify themselves with or without religion."

Then disappointment came: No editor wanted to publish the work. Noëlle had to resort to publishing it herself—finding a printer, proofing it, and having it printed. It was a huge job. Finally it was pulled off: the book came out in May 1976. There were still many errors, but it would be ready for Iyengar's visit in June. Many students bought a copy, which helped to pay off the enormous expense.

Noëlle wrote: "It is not a book for reading. Like all contemplative thought, these excerpts are to be studied and combined to form a kind of synthesis that becomes a complete education."

Georgia and Philippe LeConte
Paris, 2011

Noëlle's India Journal, 1959

I had done yoga from books, searched "everywhere," and followed different teachers for a while. I had acquired some firm beliefs and was pretty dogmatic about them. I believe that I was in a frame of mind and with similar training as many others who are about to experience the shock of meeting B.K.S. Iyengar. In these notes, I mention things that I would not say today, but they contain such freshness, such faith, such joy, that it would be a pity to correct them. I prefer to offer them as they are, with all their imperfections.

JULY 1, 1959: Phew, I am off. Papa was willing to lend me what I still needed, and just as he came to drive me to the airport, Colonel Fromji called to say that Iyengar has accepted me as his student. It looks like it is all coming together. After so many struggles, this feels good.

JULY 7: Bombay. The place buzzes with the sound of voices. Trees rustle in the light evening breeze. Pleasant town, crowded with a mass of people dressed in shades of white and color. Some are very dark-skinned. I am going to swim in the shower, after swimming in the monsoon, and after that I fear I will be swimming in my bed, it is that hot and humid!

JULY 11: As arranged, I waited for the weekend to meet Iyengar and watched him teach his class today. His students are much brighter than the ones I have seen in Europe. He does not give the impression of going easy. Although kind, he does not tolerate the halfway manner of teaching we have in Europe. Everything has to be done right, into the smallest details: *yoga*, then *bhoga* (pleasure). They teach me this word after class at the home of a student where we gather for a picnic. Very pleasant atmosphere.

JULY 13: Pune. Departure at 8:15 a.m. by fast train, which takes four hours to do 100 km and stops everywhere, even between stations. Breakfast on the train served on small trays. Arrival in Pune: Porters dressed in red hang from the windows even before the train comes to a standstill. There are at least two coolies per person! Mrs. Homji awaits me at one end of the quay, Mr. Iyengar at the other. How kind he is! He was afraid that I would feel completely lost, and since no one in his family speaks English, he came to meet me himself. When he was sure that Mrs. Homji was there to take care of me, he left, after a time was arranged for my first lesson the next morning.

JULY 14: First lesson with Iyengar. I am dead but very interested. If I last, I will get extremely healthy and exchange all my cellulite for muscle.

JULY 15: I am as dead today as yesterday; this girl is bushed.

JULY 16: More and more worn out.

JULY 17: On my way to Iyengar's house in the bus, I got off a stop too early. Somebody took me to Iyengar. The next day he sent his son to the stop to wait for me.

July 18: No class, phew. Iyengar is in Bombay.

July 20: I take advantage of the opportunity to write my parents. "Iyengar is marvelous: he was kind enough to meet me at the station. He is also a fantastic teacher, but his style of teaching is very hard at first. Exactly the opposite of everything I have been able to do in Paris and in Switzerland. We improve a pose for a long time, with all muscles in extension. Believe me, he sees all and lets you know that you just relaxed a tiny little muscle in the big toe of the left foot while he was adjusting your right knee. No relaxation between asanas. I have told myself: this kills me or it will revive me—there is no middle ground. This morning after two days off and still feeling exhausted, I had the pleasant surprise to realize that all was well and that I was gaining strength. In five lessons, he already made me improve like crazy. He is aware that he is asking too much of me, but since I told him that I already teach yoga, he trains me to teach—and that in two months! He truly tries to give me the best of himself in concentrated form, to "help all the French" indirectly through me, as he says so kindly. So far I have found in all this just a marvelous kind of gymnastics that leaves nothing untouched, because one must arrive at an interior unity. He is truly the most passionate teacher I have met till now, exactly what I need. He is going to have me change hotels so that I get better food. He says: "Careful with your health. You have come here to study, not to get sick."

July 20: From my notebook. Finally back to class. We had a great conversation. I told someone, who repeated it to Iyengar, that I was looking for a spiritual yoga. He explained that this does not exist because yoga is unity and that I cannot do anything with a weak body. And that attention means concentration. And that meditation is the moment when, after complete concentration to get a perfect pose, you hold it. That is to say, you work it.

There is a moment of such intense focus that you lose the awareness of "I." For him, each pose is a meditation, an experience of unity without sense of time, gender, or nationality. You forget everything not because you want to but because that kind of concentration forces you to.

I am back to normal, I am stronger, and in five lessons he has made me improve enormously. He has a lot of expectations for my two months. He watches everything and lets nothing escape his attention. Today we worked one hour and fifteen minutes without fatigue.

I attended his class for children (ten to sixteen years old): he leaves not a moment of respite and instead of resting assigns them (so-called) restorative poses. He links together different poses and asks such muscular effort! But the children don't seem tired; he leads them on for a long time. He has such strength, it becomes acrobatic.

July 22: Iyengar is quite satisfied; he finds that I work hard. I make a lot of progress, and my muscles hurt less. When I do Headstand, it begins to feel light.

July 23: Iyengar insists on the fact that with your students you should never go at the speed he goes with me or tire them as much, or you will lose them, for they are not courageous enough. Little by little, I realize how well he knows his art. He shows me all the preparatory steps for the most difficult asana in each group. He points out each muscle that must work, where to place my weight, where to relax, or turn, and which goal is to be reached. He is firm like a whip and beaming and affectionate when you give it your all. He helps and supports and lets go just at the moment when you cry uncle. You feel that he knows exactly how far you can go today and prepares gently for tomorrow. Today I have done Sirsasana by myself, legs firm. Strength begins to come; it is less punishing.

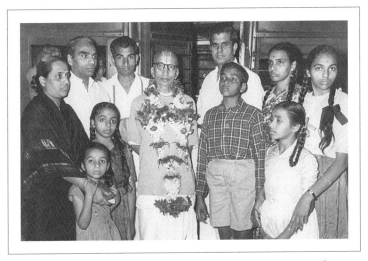

IYENGAR AND HIS FAMILY GREET KRISHNAMACHARYA, PUNE, 1961

He remains in an affectionate relationship with his Guru, Krishnama-charya and writes him everything about his work.

With the book of Yesudian in mind, I ask him if it is true that certain people can have a conversation from afar. He is somewhat skeptical and says: "How can you be sure that it is a message from the Guru?" But he does add that his letters cross with the answers of his Guru.

I really have the impression that I am in the right gear with my work, and if I meet his expectations I think he will not abandon me. He seems to know just how far he can take me and explains that it is not important if I don't know the names of muscles, because I will have a practical knowledge of them.

JULY 24: Two hours of class! I am dead but less and less stiff. He is so happy that it gives me pleasure and makes up for all the suffering I endure. Our friendship deepens: I begin to discover his simple soul, so deep. His wisdom is very human, full of experience of life and suffering. He says, "You must invite suffering so that you become friends with others who suffer." He also says that by working carefully, your intuition will develop, but that you should not seek it.

Iyengar is more and more awe-inspiring. He has something of the old sages of the past, who wait to see who you are and then give you their all. At first he made me do a lot of physical work, without going in depth. Now, our friendship deepens gradually, and with great joy I realize that I was already on his path. He is a simple man, absolutely sure of the direction in which he leads you, who has suffered the worst torments from other yogis and doctors but wordlessly survived it all due to the conviction of his work and the depth of his wisdom, which is not at all bookish, oh no!—full of life, good sense, and affection. He could be in the U.S. or at least in Bombay and earn a fortune (in the U.S. he was offered a bridge of gold). No, he prefers to stay here, to lead the simple life he has always led, surrounded by his wife and six children, who are adorable and simple like he is.

JULY 25: He is in Bombay and I work alone. God, it is difficult. I don't feel the energy running through my bloodstream yet. I read his articles, which he left me before taking off. He is truly possessed with his art; it is his great love.

JULY 31: In a letter. With the money I saved, I now go to Bombay every weekend to get two more classes and put a little spice in my life. This will allow me to visit other yoga schools, now that Iyengar has given me permission to do so.

AUGUST 5: It's still not going well. I don't have the strength to work, even though Iyengar is satisfied with the results and a little worried about me:

"Don't get sick, we have too much work to do!" He has me taken care of with lemon juice in ice cold water, no sugar, and with sparkling lemonade. It is a purge: a mix of citric acid, poison, perfume, saccharin, but I think that due to this explosive mix I am a bit better.

AUGUST 10: In a letter. Last weekend in Bombay, I saw another yoga teacher trained by the same master as Iyengar and even at the same time. No comparison—as if the same seed sown in two different plots can yield one extraordinary man from every point of view and a mediocre one from every point of view, except for the same friendliness that is characteristic of all southerners. I also visited the National Yoga Institute on Marine Drive with Parsee friends who speak French. There, men and women are separate. Of course I was not able to see the men at work. The husband of my friend has gone there and came out heartbroken after seeing all those men throwing up trying to learn to cleanse their stomachs of all the good digestive juices that nature puts there. They do it with the aid of a strip of cotton that they try to swallow.

I saw four women: three in long skirts and one in a sari. That must be practical when you put your feet up in the air. The teacher was in a sari as well. Tradition preserved without intelligence is really something idiotic.

AUGUST 10: Our friendship deepens. He explains a bunch of things, beautiful and profound but in English. Between that and my fatigue, I can't remember. He told me that his Guru had planted the seed of yoga in him but that all the work was his. His Guru wanted him to get married, so he married. He shows me his photos, and I tell him: "Your wife must be proud of you!" "No. Why? Not for that."

I return to watch him teach his class to the children. He shows me all the little things to correct, adjusting the little ones very gently, the big ones firmly. To all of them, he makes it clear that they must lengthen and they must relax. He tells me: "Now you understand the philosophy? People speak of philosophy because they have read books. Philosophy is a way of life, not a study! I plant a seed in these boys, and afterwards they can either develop it or let it dry up. I don't impose my personality on them. If I did, where would be their originality? I give them a means to create themselves. When they have understood, I let the yoga do its work in them. When we work together, there is no duality. We work; each one forgets who he is, completely into his work. If one makes a mistake, it is my mistake. If he makes progress, it is my progress as well. We share the same effort and the same joy: unity is created."

AUGUST 11: He has given me a special pranayama assignment that is very stimulating: I was not able to sleep during my siesta, nor in the evening before midnight. This must be given to people who are sluggish, not the active ones.

Tomorrow morning I must be at his place at 8:45 a.m. One student can't come, so he invited me to come and watch him do his exercises. Our friend-ship intensifies; I am truly his favorite because he notices my zeal and that I don't hide my troubles. When I am tired I tell him: give me a moment, after that I try again. Or I ask *bus* (enough), and if he answers "One more minute," I stay, even if it is very hard, asking him the time every ten seconds!

AUGUST 12: Iyengar works forty minutes nonstop in front of me. It is admira-ble, not a false movement, all is precision. He does the most difficult things, not without work, but superbly, without balking at the effort. He explains that it is better to treat your body like a slave, like Maya, rather than the common way of renouncing so-called everything and remaining a slave and stunted. He reads me excerpts of the Yoga Sutra of Patanjali, where the great sage says that you arrive at self-realization through long and arduous work, without allowing a day of rest, without wearying of it, without getting discouraged despite illness, troubles, etc. He urges himself "to keep going ahead." You really get the impression that in everything he does, he tries his best to go a little farther today. He is happy with the least amount of progress because he does not seek Perfection, but the small perfections of every day. This man really radiates *joie de vivre* despite his poverty.

We speak of powers. He answers that when you realize you received a power, you must be glad about your progress but certainly not serve yourself by it. If you seek to develop this way, you become proud and get sidetracked: goodbye spiritual improvement. Then he adds: "The very great yogis can use them, because they know what is good and bad. They are sure about not using them for the worse, but this is not possible for people like you and me." What humility!

He will not accept the title of yogi. He says, "I am on the path. How can you say that you have arrived?"

Afterwards we talk about books written about yoga. He says: "Don't read, experiment. I read only when something new happens. Then I look at what Patanjali has to say about it."

I ask him if the powers that people talk about are real or symbolic. He answers that it is reality.

During Corpse Pose, I had a fright. I had the impression that life left me. I called him; I felt that he was not watching over me. He said that it was a pity to have cut it off, that it was a new experience to be faced, that what is new is frightening, but that it takes courage. We talked about an out-of-body experience. He tells me that it is very dangerous, bad for peacefulness and mental balance and counter to yoga. That it is not what will happen to me, but that I was beginning to feel the void, and that the void and solitude are always scary in the beginning. It was a very little step towards the Self.

AUGUST 16: I ask him what he thinks of all the stomach cleansing we witnessed on Marine Drive and other interior cleansing with or without a rag. He answers that it is very bad. Patanjali permits it only in rare cases. He adds that if others do it, they will invite illness. He adds that the people I saw yesterday (at another yoga school that was not great) were sickly for that reason. They teach it there to all students.

AUGUST 17: We talk about praying. He explains that he says a mantra when holding an energetic pose for a long time, but that most of the time his prayer is to serve his Lord through serving others. And truly, he serves with all his heart!

This morning I told him laughingly, "I am crazy to come from Paris to work with you!" "And I am crazy to teach you the way I am doing." "My Maman told me that only the crazy ones and the passionate ones accomplish anything in life." "I agree," he says, but adds that in his twenty-five years of teaching he only worked like this for two people: Yehudi Menuhin and me. It is because Menuhin serves the whole world with his violin. And I serve my brothers and sisters in Europe through yoga.

AUGUST 17: In a letter to Maman. You wonder about my teacher? I am more and more content with him. I now spend three hours with him every day: poses, breathing, philosophy, life. We talk about everything, except about nothing, and I marvel that all my prior evolution has led me to his path. Just like the Indian saying: "When the student is ready, the teacher shall appear." He is not there if you don't search for him, but he is put in your path. I would like to stay a long time, to pump all this wisdom that is so simple, so human and so divine at the same time. There is no telling, you don't just find God in life; I mean, God is not what the theologians say he is. He is much more profound and simple.

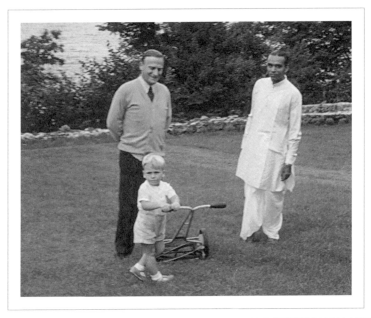

The more I learn, the more I like St. John: "He who has seen has borne witness," and St. Paul: "I know a man who was overjoyed . . . but what he has seen and understood cannot be expressed in words." Such great men can speak of God without saying nonsense. But theologians take hold of the experiences and words of the sages and argue with their heads instead of speaking from a mystical experience, which they lack. And so religion degenerates. Here I am around a sage who does not know that he is a sage, who has a wife he loves as much as a Hindu can love, meaning ten times more than us, and who has six children. They live in two rooms, in a working class neighborhood and no one, seeing him, would guess that he has already traveled to Europe twice and also to the U.S., which is extraordinary for a poor Indian.

I do wonderful things and discover, as Iyengar says, that "God has blessed me" in sending me this master, because my observations of various yoga institutes in Bombay are disappointing. He comes from a long line of Gurus. You could say that they pass on the know-how by word of mouth, which allows us to benefit from the experience of generations of yogis.

AUGUST 18: Iyengar reads me again and again passages from Patanjali, as well as from the Hatha Yoga Pradipika, which is a little later, where he insists on the fact that there is only one yoga. "There is no Raja Yoga without Hatha Yoga, and there is no Hatha Yoga without Raja Yoga." One yoga encompasses morals, poses, breathing, concentration, contemplation, integration. It is wrong to speak of physical and spiritual yoga; this is a modern distinction. Elsewhere Patanjali says: "I am going to show you summarily some poses," which means, according to Iyengar, that there are many and that he does not explain all the details, because in olden times they were passed on by the Gurus. The ancient books were written only for them.

Iyengar explains with several examples that these books are written in verse, like long poems, and that you cannot take them literally but must study them with common sense without believing in fantasy. What makes it difficult for us Westerners is that the only English translation in existence (in 1959) does not conform to the Sanskrit, and sometimes entire verses of explanatory passages are left out.

He tells me that in certain poses you lose the sense of duality, you feel a peace, an incredible, indescribable joy, and that even if you have to struggle a whole life for one second of that joy, it is worth it.

His good sense leaves you flabbergasted: he tells me that Swami X says that consciously holding the breath, with lungs either full or empty, is not essential, but unconscious retention is. He adds: how can you withhold your breath unconsciously? When you are stunned by a beautiful sunset, all thought stops, and you lose the notion of duality. But how can you go looking for such moments? If you look for them, they escape you.

We speak about how to concentrate according to different methods. He explains that if you concentrate on the forehead, or the tip of the nose, or the chest, it makes no difference. He prefers to concentrate on his chest because it is the seat of the Self. For that reason, you usually do the *Namaste* at chest level. This gesture of worship, palms open and touching, is a complex symbol as long as you have not understood the unity of everything. It means: my soul and the Universal Soul are one, or my soul and your soul are one—it is all the same thing.

Regarding physical and spiritual yoga, he says: "When you realize that without breath there is no life, you feel gratitude towards God, who gives life through breath. When you give up your life to God during the exhale and receive your life from God during the inhale, where is the physical yoga? All during pranayama, you give yourself to this meditation."

Regarding the rules of morality in various communities, he says that you have to do your best. Keep in mind that you cannot advance spiritually without some framework, whatever it is. He is so solid and radiates peace and joy!

AUGUST 19: He never accepts what you achieved as definitive: if you can do that, then try to go a little bit further. And so you always suffer, because you always go further, but must realize that you are making incredible progress very quickly. This morning he was excited about my improvement: I am really happy, he said in English. "Fully happy. That is my way of teaching!"

AUGUST 20: I collapse in tears doing Kurmasana (Tortoise), I suffer that much. He consoles me and caresses my cheek: "Why did you not tell me?

Why are you worried? You are making progress!" I answer that I am not worried, that I simply hurt a lot, and I put him at ease: "Don't worry about my tears, I think that my nerves are giving up, but continue, I am very happy."

It is rare to find a man so firm and so tender at the same time. He is truly in the service of the God in you. He is always there when you need something, always ready to help if you weaken, always ready to help as long as you make an effort, even if your strength fails you. Love is truly and plainly incarnate in him and an intelligent love.

August 24: I return again to watch him teach the boys. He is great, full of action and youth. On the way out, he explains that if you are diligent, your conscience dictates that you "try to go further," even when everyone thinks it is perfect. You have to go from the gross to the subtle, from skin to bone, always further. The whole nervous system must work, and that can only happen in a total extension (without tension), all through the flesh. That is creative work, and there you have the spiritual work: through the nerves, you touch the subtle body.

You have to admit that being able to do what I do while my digestion is in such a mess shows that yoga must invigorate me: my teeth are whiter, and the whites of my nails look bigger.

August 26: Still no period. The red patch on my belly has disappeared, and the one on my arm is getting smaller. This morning I have swollen glands in my left groin and by evening another painful but smaller one on the right.

August 27: Fantastic lesson. The dose is increased to a level of red alert, and it works, phew, finally. In fact, I am not tired. He is happy and tells me that

I exceeded his expectations. I just slept half an hour before lunch and woke up ready to begin again. I have aches that won't quit, in my back, ribs—and let's not even talk about my legs.

He told me: "Don't hesitate to write when you have the least bit of doubt about your students, good or bad, and I will answer."

AUGUST 27: In a letter to my family. Goodness gracious, what a way to work! Yesterday and today I did two hours of asana at a stretch. I am beginning to hold up! But the Monday after coming back from Bombay, I couldn't do a thing. I let him turn me in all directions, just saying *bus* (enough) when I feel that he exaggerates. This does not keep him from continuing when he thinks I am soft, but generally he stops when it is really too much. He has an incredible flair for knowing.

The medications you sent did me good and let me have three great sessions. He praised me more than ever and told me that I exceeded his highest expectations, how about that? You grumble about my belly, but that's nothing my dears. Remember that the liver and a headache go together for me? You can imagine what it was like when the smallest effort felt like a hammer blow to my temples and my head felt squeezed in a vise the rest of the time. But that's not all: I don't have a single muscle, a single joint, rib, or vertebra that does not hurt. That is the ransom for my progress. Fortunately he informs me that "Tomorrow it will be worse, and after that it will begin to ease up." So I trust him and don't worry.

When his oldest daughter, Geeta, saw that a woman from overseas had come to work with her father, Geeta brought her blanket and really began to work. This morning he had me work with her. She is like rubber—ah, youth! He does not push her so that she does not turn against the work— ah, Indian astuteness. Besides, that would risk hindering her growth; she is only fourteen. It is a matter of getting her interest piqued and preserving her flexibility; when she becomes stronger, it will be perfect.

AUGUST 31: Always make an effort with the lungs empty to prevent palpitations and stress on the heart.

SEPTEMBER 1: Today I am very tired. A very good class because he does everything. He shows me that in the Hatha Yoga Pradipika it says that Raja Yoga and samadhi are the same thing. Raja Yoga is not a means but an end, just about. It is not an approach but the goal you want to reach: the mystical union. He tells me that in every pose you have to discover yoga as Patanjali defined it.

Here is a man who truly understands that God is One and that as long as you divide and subdivide, the Goal eludes you. In all his seeking his focus is on Unity, not union but Unity. He is full of zeal in his quest for this Goal. "The moral, physical and mental all must work together; then no duality remains and the Spirit is there. When the spirit no longer obstructs, the Spirit or Supreme Soul is free and Is." You move from the known to the Unknown, from the spirit to the Spirit.

He tells me that he suffered for four years as I do, but that now he savors the fruit. However, one day when "the body refused," as he said, I saw him play a record for fifteen minutes to allow him to hold a pose while getting some distraction from the pain. When he got up, he was sweating. He does not seem to get the fruit every day! But he can work an hour or two and do the most difficult things without getting tired. His body is now truly his friend. Once he told the boys: "The strength of will is in the buttocks. If you can squeeze those muscles, if they are strong, you have the force of will."

This man radiates peace, purity, stability, even though he lives from day to day, without money in reserve. He is solid as a rock. You could apply to him the verse of the psalm "the zeal of Thy House devours me" or "You are a rock and upon that rock shall I build my church."

Today I was tired, and he scolded me. "You don't work for yourself; you have taken on a heavy responsibility. You work for others. I know that from now on you will be a first-class teacher, with all I have taught you. But that is not enough, I want more. Be strong, get up, let's go." How can you resist such drive?

One day I told him that I thought that *Ha-tha* could also mean the union of the sympathetic and parasympathetic nervous system, with one working during the day and the other at night. He said: "Yes, also—it could be a lot of things."

SEPTEMBER 2: I have a stomach full of air! Even so, we make progress in every way. He is overjoyed. "Imagine how it could be if you were feeling well?" To encourage me, he says that I did Kurmasana (Tortoise Pose) just like him. Yes, sure, but he forgets that he does it alone, while I am helped quite a bit.

In a letter to Papa: Some days I measure 3 to 4 centimeters extra around my waist, that's how much air I have in my stomach. Despite everything, we work like madmen. He is excited about my courage and my capacity for work, and I about everything that comes from him. He did not think he could get me this far, push me this much. Only a short month of work left. If I could have eaten better, I would have had more resistance, and I would have been able to go farther. I will have to come back another time with mom, so she can feed "her baby" properly. My vacation has been fantastic, despite all my health problems. There are wonderful people in the world, and it is a joy to become their friend, even at the expense of taking it easy!

In a letter to my sister: I am going to skip the end of my trip when I had planned to visit some interesting places. I prefer to come back. I have so much to learn from him. But I will go to Bombay every weekend. Last weekend in September, I will leave for home directly from Bombay. It is less expensive and less tiring and will give me a few extra days with you to teach you all I can of what I have learned here.

I don't need any more medications, thanks. I have enough until I leave. What I have serves its purpose, and when things get too bad Mother Nature does her job and redelivers everything the same way it entered. After that I feel better. Despite that, everything is okay. The asana and breathing have their effect. I have enough energy to work, and when I am mush he does the work for me. Don't worry, I don't look bad. He and his wife look after me with maternal tenderness.

It is really amazing to see the detachment and generosity of this man. The more I work, the more I advance, and the happier he is. I believe that if I would pass him by one day, he would be overjoyed, but thank God, he will always be a hundred leagues ahead to pull me along! He is a true Guru, like you dream of meeting one day but rarely do. I have an unforgettable opportunity. He is a man who has understood life. He does his job as best he can, no excuses, aware of his weaknesses and trying to correct them, knowing that it takes time and being very simple and submitting to the Lord. Never totally satisfied, he ever tries to do better and tells me about his discoveries with childlike pleasure. He does not act the perfect and irreproachable teacher. This way he is near to us, he is one of us and can take us in his wake. He is the Lord incarnate.

SEPTEMBER 6: In Bombay. I got a sprain in the left thoracic area, under my shoulder blade. It hurts something awful, even lying down, but what is marvelous and unforgettable is the attitude of Iyengar. It started with a little grating noise next to the spine in Sarvangasana. Since it did not hurt, I continued with Halasana and then began to feel some pain. By chance he was next to me, and I told him, as I often did, that I had a pain and exactly

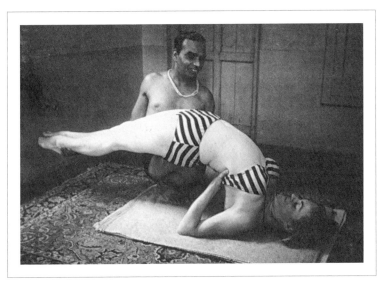

IYENGAR WITH NOËLLE IN PARSVA SARVANGASANA

where. He said: "Quick, stop." It seemed strange to be gentle with me; normally he would say "I know, I know, go on." We retry the pose, impossible. He touches my back and says, "It must be there, and that is a sprain." It was exactly the right spot. We try standing poses, impossible. Then he lets me relax and continues his class, but it was terrible, and I could not breathe. I was close to giving up and thought, "This is all I need."

After a moment he came close and said, "Standing poses." I thought, "This is crazy," but I got up and tried. I couldn't even lift my left arm to a straight angle. But he came, pushed against my back, pulled here, pushed there, and it went better. Second pose, same thing, and after that he took the initiative: this pose, not that one but the other. Then he said, "Now twists." Again I thought he is crazy, if only he would leave me alone and let me rest. And we did simple twists, then the others. Next we did the forward bends and he told me, "Now the Wheel." "Oh, no!" "Why not?" Because it went better all the time and he had been right about all the other things, I tried the Wheel at first from a standing position, and he helped a lot. Next we did the ones beginning from a lying down position, but it was very hard. After that, Pigeon, and finally he said, "*Bus.*" But I could have gone on; it was much better. Afterwards my friends came to pick me up, and I was able to last the whole afternoon without saying anything and without them noticing.

SEPTEMBER 7: My sprain is better, but I am tired. I did not sleep well.

SEPTEMBER 8: The sprain is almost forgotten, but Iyengar is very attentive, and it is a good pretext to make a little less effort. During the afternoon, we study the photos that he had made for me and the descriptions that go with them. It is clear, well written, all in good order, and nothing missing. What precision for an Indian, even for a French person.

SEPTEMBER 9: A very good class. The sprain seems better except when I go deep into Sarvangasana. Iyengar tells me that he had me do it again right away, but that you should not do that with anyone; rather let it rest for five or six days. But we have no time to lose to let me rest. If this happens with other students, it is better to do only standing poses.

Again about physical and spiritual yoga: eyes open symbolizes consciousness in Eastern stories. (The eyes of statues are opened symbolically at the time of a ceremony when God is asked to take possession of this new body.) It seems to me that the Apocalypse also contains a story of open eyes symbolizing consciousness. He tells me the story of two men who are in a forest. The first one, who has eyes but no limbs, says to the other, who has limbs but is blind, "There is a fire in the forest, and it is getting closer. It is going to destroy both of us. Carry me on your back, and I will show you the way. Please carry me so we can both save our lives." Iyengar continues: "How can you say that the one yoga is inferior to the other? Both are necessary."

He also tells me a story from the Upanishads, about two birds. One sits motionless in the top of a tree, and the other tastes any fruit he can find on his way up to meet the first bird. Of these fruits, some are bitter, some good, but he tries everything and goes from experience to experience without stopping. He reaches the top of the tree and then forgets everything and stays there. "How can you say that one way is better than the other if both reached the same point?"

SEPTEMBER 10: He asks if I have done my breathing practice this morning. I tell him no. He is sad and insists: "Please do it," but does not scold me. I don't want to deceive him, but I can't be bothered, and one is forever disturbed in this darned country where privacy is nonexistent.

He walks me home, holding his bike—remarkable! He asks if I know what the Trinity is. I know what I learned at Catholic school and from theology classes, but in case he has something else to teach me I feign ignorance. He begins an unforgettable explanation of three in one and one in three, in all its forms and details, with examples from everyone's daily life. Because he has thought about it so much, everything seems simple when it passes through his soul! Body, mind, and spirit—action, intelligence, and love. He also talks about the joy of patience—to me who is always impatient, pressed for time.

We arrive, and he stays for a visit. We chat for two unforgettable hours. He tells me about his life, his experiences, that he cannot do without his exercises and that to him it is no longer work but a passion. I assure him that for me it is still a chore. He tells me not to worry, it will come. He talks about prayer in pranayama. I tell him that it is a big effort for me and that I cannot really concentrate enough for it to become a prayer. He says, "You will need several years."

He is deeply religious. "Everything is sent me by my Lord," he says. "I give myself to Him, worship Him, and give Him all I can, gratefully." He continues: "People say that peace of mind is an end. No, it is a beginning. I have arrived at that point and can explain everything up to there. Now I struggle to discover what comes after. But this peace of mind is not an end in itself; it is a beginning as well as a means, an instrument."

He goes on: "You should never criticize a colleague. When a student comes from another teacher, he must create his own experience: Try it this way; what do you feel? Is it better? No more pain? Personal experience is the only real approach." He tells me the story of the donkey taken to market by a father and son. The son is disturbed by criticism, but the father continues on his way. "Don't let anyone bother you. You must find your own way. You must arrive at a level of maturity that makes you sure of yourself in the midst of everyone's criticism."

SEPTEMBER 11: In photo session. Yesterday we took it easier, trying to be less achy for today. Iyengar is charming and the photographer very slow. We killed ourselves holding a pose until he deigned to push the clicker. Iyengar helps me as much as possible. He takes my place while the photographer measures the light, and he avoids any unnecessary effort. I do what I can, but my muscles are not warmed up. It's okay but not the best. I hoped that he would always stay by my side for the poses, because I see the difference clearly and realize the progress I must make. But he prefers me alone so that I can show the pictures to my students.

SEPTEMBER 15: Letter to Maman. My departure is set; I will arrive September 28. Don't worry, I am still whole and I walk with my head held high, because my teacher is maybe the only Indian around who has his feet on the ground in the sense of philosophy. I say that of course because we have more or less the same ideas, which I discovered with incredible pleasure. Spiritually he could be my father, and he is a little bit, because all alone I had gone as far as I could. But physically he is not at all like my father: my joints are in too bad a shape to assume that honor.

SEPTEMBER 15: Letter to Papa. This morning I had my lesson at the same time as the oldest daughter of Iyengar, who works very well. She has progressed tremendously since July and begins to want to teach, to the great joy of her father. My visit will at the least have this as a result. The whole family has adopted me, one being nicer than the other.

SEPTEMBER 20: Got up at 6 a.m., took two buses, class at 8:15 a.m.! Very good class, despite feeling tired and lacking sleep. When I cannot get the Headstand, Iyengar tells everyone: "Isn't this surprising. She has not slept enough." Me: "How do you know?" "Her eyes are red." It is extraordinary how he pays attention to everything. He sees right away that my friend from Bombay, Kaushi, gave me some new toe-rings.

SEPTEMBER 21: In the boys' class. Iyengar wants me to teach it so he can correct me, but I don't accept. I don't know their language or the Sanskrit name of all the asanas, and I cannot be as energetic as he is with them, which is important with boys. If he had not come, I would have felt ready to face it, but him being there . . .

Afterwards he accompanies me to Main Street. He tells me lots of things, such as: perfect women do not reincarnate into men, but are canonized in his religion as well.

He tells me that Krishna says in the Gita: "The eyes of mortals cannot see me. I am going to give you special eyes." (This brings to mind St. Paul, speaking in Damascus!) Arjuna becomes blind and then asks for his mortal eyes back because he cannot tolerate that special vision. Iyengar continues: Shankaracharya says that Self-realization is granted only a very small number of people. The others must visualize God as their Lord. In India a feminine personification of God exists as well. The same Shankaracharya has composed long verses to her that are still read in the temples today. Cows can only visualize the Lord as a Cow, and man can only visualize him as a Man. This is an indispensable steppingstone, which you cannot reject on the basis of philosophy.

Then—all the while walking along in the street—he points out that I am not Noëlle but that Noëlle is a label. I am something that they call here the Self, with a capital S, which you could translate probably with the word Soul, provided that you don't differentiate between the universal Soul, the unborn Soul, and what the Christians call the soul with a small s. But I am not what I believe I am, which is all that is implied with the pronouns I, me, myself. Here those names are designated for the self with a small s. The task is to realize that you are not the small but the large S and to pass from the one to the other, detaching from the first and merging into Unity.

Just as we cannot know who our parents are if we are not told, we cannot know who God is. We have to create an image of him that becomes clearer with time and that enables us to reach Him in steps, as if climbing a ladder.

September 23: I will be leaving soon. Iyengar has found me a reasonable translation of the Hatha Yoga Pradipika, which he gives me with a kind dedication.

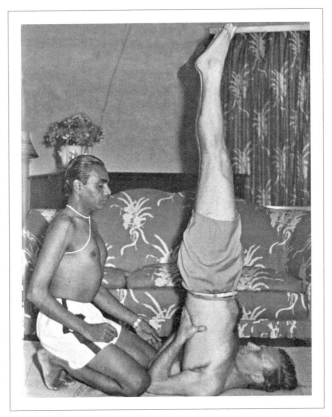

IYENGAR ADJUSTS YEHUDI MENUHIN IN SARVANGASANA, GSTAAD, 1956

SEPTEMBER 24: I was so sore that to help me relax at the end of class he put on some records. The first is one of his conferences, which I could not understand at all. I no longer want to make the effort, and English is still difficult for me. Next are songs by J. Douai to make me feel "at home." And finally a concert for violin and orchestra by Beethoven played by Yehudi Menuhin, who seems to caress or embrace his violin.

At a reception at Iyengar's home in honor of my leaving, Iyengar gives me a small bottle of sandalwood oil and, for protection of my ears on the Vespa (an Italian scooter), a very pretty, "typically Indian" scarf, handmade in the villages. All the girls gather around me to do my hair like theirs. Geeta has a hard time with my hair, which is not oiled and so fine that it slips away each time she wants to do something. Her hands touch so gently that I hardly feel them. Then they drape me in a black sari belonging to their maman. When Iyengar returns and sees me, he is very happy. "How small you look in a sari," he says. Geeta and her mother prepare lunch while I play with the little ones, who have taken me into their new upstairs room, where I see a portrait of their father and family photo albums.

For each person, there is a slightly raised board serving as a seat, and in front of it is a large plate with two small cups. Next to the plate, a tumbler of water: the table is set. I am given the place of honor, opposite Iyengar. His wife does not sit down; she serves the whole time and will eat at the end, when everyone is finished. Then Geeta will serve her, and she can eat in peace. It is the same ritual as we have on the farms in the French countryside. It seems to me more relaxing for the hostess, so that she does not have to get up all the time.

They have put a mix of rice on my plate with peas plus other things I don't recognize. Next to that are milk curds with cucumber, green beans with rice, sweet rice mixed with a bunch of tasty things, a chapatti and two small apple fritters, and I don't know what else. You eat in the order you want and ask for more of what you like, and whenever there is room on the plate, they put something different. In one of the small cups is a sweet liquid, delicious and warm, but what is it? No idea!

You eat with your fingers, very neatly (except for me, but Iyengar comes to my aid and asks for a spoon). This way of eating seems to me quite hygienic.

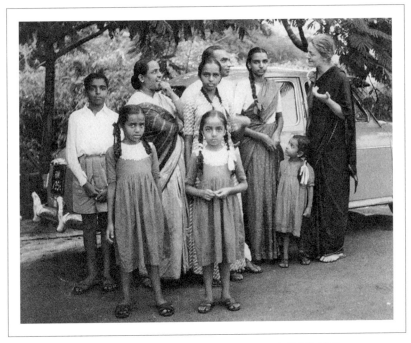

NOËLLE WITH B.K.S. IYENGAR AND HIS FAMILY, PUNE, 1959

After all, if my hand is poorly washed it is just my own perspiration and not saliva left by others, as could be the case when you eat with a fork, as we do. At any rate, they have us wash our hands before the meal and also after, and you eat with just three fingers of the right hand: thumb, index finger, and middle finger. These customs are characteristic of different communities.

I have begun to sit in tailor fashion (Svastikasana), like Iyengar. Later during the meal, he mentions that I am the only woman sitting like that. The women always keep one knee up to hide their face when a man enters the room. The right knee is on the floor, the left one in the air, with the left hand placed on the left foot. He tells me the significance of all these details with such patience.

While Mrs. Iyengar is changing, the girls take me to the sun-bathed terrace to show me the view. I cannot stay put because the cement floor burns my feet, which naturally are bare; they don't wear sandals here except for going out, and even then not always. All these little feet already have thick skin underneath; mine seem so silly next to theirs.

After that, the whole group goes to the zoo. The weather seems more or less improved after yesterday's big storm. We look at quite a few animals and suddenly, like a flash, the storm is back. That gives cause for lots of laughter, fun, and games, like moving your ears or your nose, making different sounds with your mouth, etc. We take pictures and hope they will come out.

SEPTEMBER 25: Very good class despite all the soreness from yesterday. He makes me link together an incredible number of Wheel Poses, arching back from standing while he supports me. The first ones were so difficult with all my aches that I could not even let my arms drop. After that it got better. Poor Iyengar was dead from having to carry a weight like mine. He said laughingly: "This is the first time I perspire doing the Wheel Pose!"

SEPTEMBER 27: Class in Bombay. Iyengar brings the photos from Thursday, taken with the whole family. It is our last class. We take him back to the station. He jokes the whole way, not wanting to become emotional. The train takes off, and from the door opening he calls: "Tell your mother that I send you back whole, not in pieces." Burst of laughter, big arm movements, and he is gone. What unforgettable joy, what an extraordinary stay, but how happy I am to go home. I was afraid not to last till the end; I am at the end of my rope. He felt it and did all he could to help me not to fail.

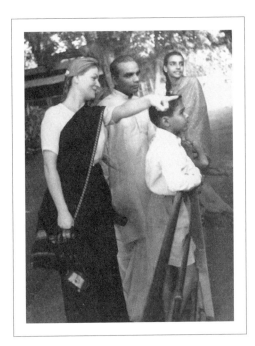

Sparks of Divinity 1959–1975

✳

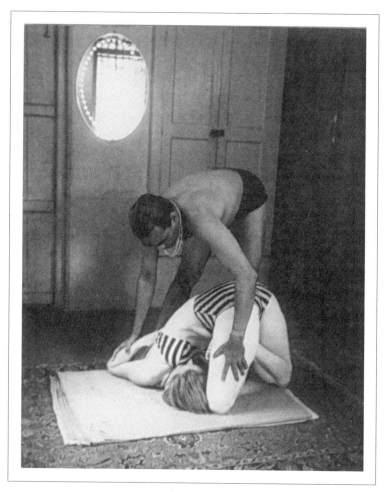

IYENGAR WITH NOËLLE IN PARSVA PINDASANA

1959

1.1. Enjoy all you do; then you feel you are free from the self.

1.2. I am always happy with the smallest improvement. I do not try to reach Perfection but only the little perfection of every day.

1.3. Will power develops by regular discipline.

1.4. There is only one yoga that includes morals, asana, pranayama, concentration, contemplation, integration. It is wrong to speak of physical yoga and of spiritual yoga; it is a modern discrimination; neither Patanjali nor the Hatha Yoga Pradipika speaks of it.

1.5. Do the work today and do not leave it for tomorrow; that can never solve anything, but adds anxieties.

1.6. Spiritual yoga does not exist. Yoga is unity, and it is impossible to do something with a weak body.

1.7. Please convey my best wishes to all your pupils and please tell them that hard work alone brings results, and not half-hearted effort.

1.8. People speak about philosophy because they have read books. Philosophy is a way of living, not something to study.

1.9. If a man is old, give him neck balance and ask him to do pranayama with the nostrils, slowly and deeply. Then he will get peace of mind.

1.10. A patient approach will bring much knowledge.

1.11. Yoga is circulation: by stretching, blood arrives, the thick blood is driven back, the energy goes on to feed the nerves. Little by little, intuition improves, but do not try to find it.

1.12. When you say, "It is bad," you close the pupil's mind instead of correcting it. You have to take what the pupil brings and from that pull something better.

1.13. Never criticize a colleague; when a pupil comes we have to first let him do by his own experience. Then say, "Now try this way. What do you feel? Is it better? Worse?" Personal experience is the only way to approach a subject.

1.14. When *pratyahara* comes about, it all happens at the same time. Even in ordinary life, if for example you are absorbed in a book, complete unification happens sometimes; similarly with a posture. But this is only the very beginning of *samadhi*. True samadhi comes when one can stay for a long while in that state, engulfed by God. Joy also comes after that, in true samadhi. What you should look for is unification in all the postures, in all your acts; that is integration.

1.15. In my book, I divided the body into three parts: the head: yoga of knowledge; the chest: yoga of love; the limbs: yoga of action. How can you say that one is higher and the other lower? These three parts make a whole.

1.16. Never think of yesterday. If things go well, look for the coming joy. If you feel that you are wrong, only then go back. Not otherwise.

1.17. You should be like a farmer: the day he sows, he is happy not because he is thinking of the future harvest; he is happy to have made a beautiful planting and to have sown well. The day the first leaf arises, he is happy with the little leaf; the day there are ten of them, he is happy with the ten leaves, but he is not happy because he is thinking of the fruits; he does not know exactly what they will be like. It is the same for us: we know that one day we may realize ourselves, but it will happen when God blesses us.

1.18. Invite suffering; then you will make friends with those who suffer.

1.19. When we are aware of the fact that without breathing there is no life, we feel very grateful to God, who gives life through breathing. We surrender our life to God during exhalation, and we receive our life from God during inhalation. As long as we do pranayama, we surrender ourselves to this meditation. Where is the difference between physical and spiritual yoga?

1.20. Do not accept what you attained as something definitive. If you can do that, then try to go further.

1.21. The eight steps of yoga: *Yama* and *niyama* are the ethical methods within (individual) and without (social). *Asana* and *pranayama* are for perfecting the physical body. Pranayama and *pratyahara* are for control of the mind and senses. *Dharana, dhyana,* and *samadhi* are for realization of the Self.

1.22. Will power is here (*he gives a slap on a young man's buttocks*). If you know how to contract the muscles, if they are strong, you get will power.

1.23. I am not a yogi, I am on the path. How can anybody say he has arrived?

1.24. Don't go to bed with tomorrow's pressure of work. Whatever you have to do, you have to do it, so why worry about the matter?

1.25. Sleep is a necessity. Relaxed sleep is far superior to tense or anxious sleep. A short, relaxed sleep period is sufficient to refresh one quickly.

1.26. Please, do the postures yourself while you are explaining them to your pupils. That will keep you in touch. Never miss Sirsasana, Sarvangasana, and pranayama. Never say you have no time for your practices. Take my example: you know how hard I work, yet you know how I keep in touch without missing a day. Do not think about having no time; then you will squeeze the time for your practices.

1.27. How can a tree know it gives shade and that its shade is good? How can you know at which height you are? Go on!

1.28. When we work together, there is no duality: we work. Each one forgets who he is. He is completely in his work. If someone makes a mistake, it is my fault. If he makes progress, it is my progress. We share the same effort, the same joy: unity is created.

1.29. There are five senses but: the mind governs the senses. Breathing governs the mind. The nerves govern breathing. The asana give control over the nerves. When the mind is stabilized, then character can improve and personalize itself.

1.30. In some postures, we lose the sense of duality and we live in peace, in a joy we cannot express in words. And even if we have to fight all our life to find this joy once more, it is worth doing it.

1.31. In yoga, if the stretch is not complete, there is no unity of body, mind, and spirit. So also in relaxation.

1.32. I know that people, whether from the East or West, need rest and relaxation. Whether people are from the East or West, the tensions are there. Tensions are not stretches. If the stretching is good, relaxation is bound to be complete. A half-hearted stretch gives a half-hearted relaxation.

1.33. In asana also, maintain a detached attitude to the body, and at the same time, do not neglect to stretch fully. Rushing at things saps the strength. Whether you are in India or Paris, the mind should be calm, and everything should be done in rhythm.

1.34. Even when everyone thinks it is perfect, if you are conscientious, your conscience says, "Try to get further."

1.35. Peace of mind does not come by varying the methods of pranayama. Let them stick to one method for a long time.

1.36. Sometimes the body says, "Yes," and the mind says, "Excuse me today." Sometimes the mind says, "Yes," and the body, "Excuse me." I always say, "Let us go ahead."

1.37. You should always do a little bit more than you can, in quality and in quantity.

1.38. There is no spiritual improvement without an ethical framework.

1.39. Never consider pranayama as an exercise, but as a prayer. Breathing is life.

1.40. Have divine feelings while teaching, talking, resting, and even in sleep. Go to bed surrendering your day's work to the Lord. While getting up, pray and have Him in your heart to give you strength and determination to carry out the day's work.

1.41. May the Lord guide you throughout your practices. Surrender to Him, and He will look after your comforts.

1.42. You are ever in my thoughts. I can only pray the Lord to keep you always yoga-minded.

1.43. Purging the body and mind with persistent practice, and nonattachment to things which occur directly or indirectly, leads you to the light of knowledge that reveals the Truth of oneness and everlasting peace, which cannot be written in words but experienced only.

1.44. As a teacher, you have taken on a heavy responsibility. You do not work for yourself alone. You must study for the benefit of others. Even when you are tired, keep up your courage. You can do no less. I want no more.

1.45. When the mind is no more a screen, the Soul (*Atma*) is free and shines as pure crystal with no reflection on it. When the Self is free from the contact of things, that is the state of experiencing *samadhi*.

1.46. Often I say some *mantram* to help me remain in a pose, but the principle of my prayer is to serve my Lord by serving my neighbor.

1.47. All is sent by my Lord. I surrender to him, I worship him and give back to him all that I can very thankfully.

1.48. Mind, spirit, and body should be one: three in one, and one in three.

1.49. The human being is divided into five: the physical, the physiological, the psychological (the mind), the intellect, the spiritual. There is no spiritual joy (*ananda*) unless all is united and happy.

1.50. Meditation is oneness, when there is no longer time, sex, or country. The moment when, after you have concentrated on doing a pose (or anything else) perfectly, you hold it and then forget everything, not because you want to forget but because you are concentrated: this is meditation.

1.51. Regarding yourself, do not say that you are disappointed. Find time every day to do something to maintain your asana practice. Sometimes both body and mind yield to will power, and at other times they rebel. Patient and disciplined practice will bring the required will power. Even Patanjali said that yoga is mastered only by long, persistent, nonstop practice, with zeal and determination. Do not bother about failures. Failures in life lead to determination and a philosophical approach to life.

1.52. Regarding pranayama, you are like me. For years, I used to get up early to do pranayama. As soon as I did three or four minutes, I used to feel it was too much and ended the day's pranayama. It is the nature of one who has more dynamism to prefer asana, and some have life to do pranayama. After fifteen years of this irregular pranayama practice, now I find the will to do it. Even one hour at a stretch is too little now for me. This I gained patiently. I give you the same advice. Every day do five or ten minutes, even if it bores you. Then you conquer the monotony, and you will succeed. As there are no variations in pranayama, it bores. You will succeed at the end of two or three years' regular practice. Even if you do only five minutes, do it with full devotion and be one with it. You will rise up.

1.53. I plant in these boys the seed of yoga. It is for them to make the plant grow. I never force on them my personality, for then where would be their originality? I provide for them a means to become creative. When they understand this, I leave yoga to do its own work through them.

1.54. Help those who come to you. With faith in God, you will succeed.

1.55. People say that steadiness of mind is an end; no, it is a beginning. I am there; I can explain everything up to that point. Then I struggle to discover what comes after, so this steadiness is not an end, it is the beginning and the instrument.

1.56. In each posture, in each action, you should be able to find yoga in its integrity according to Patanjali's explanations:

YAMA

Satya = truth. If you do what you are doing thoroughly, it is truth toward yourself and the pose.

Brahmacharya = no loss of energy. If your mind is wandering, energy is lost. If you steady your mind, then concentration starts and energy develops inside yourself.

Aparigraha = nonpossession. You should not do the pose to possess it, but for itself, to master it, to make friends with your body in the service of God.

Ahimsa = not to harm. You should not do violence, but you should make yourself supple.

NIYAMA

Then joy comes.

Internal purity is created by purification of the nerves; external purity is there when we do not let the mind wander.

Tapas = austerity. It is difficult, but we keep the will awake for the time we have decided to do the pose.

Svadhyaya = self-development. No explanation is required.

Ishvara pranidhana = to think all the time of the divine. Finally we forget the posture; we just "are" and discover the Self within ourselves.

Pranayama

In each posture there is a special breathing and often a retention.

Pratyahara

If we are thoroughly in what we are doing, a time comes when we forget everything around us.

Dharana

Re-embrace. It is to hang on to concentration even more deeply, and in unity.

Dhyana

Firmness, stability, not to move, not to shake; this is valid for the mind as well.

Samadhi

Sometimes we enjoy a bliss that is a taste of *samadhi*—total joy, total fulfillment, unity rediscovered.

1960

2.1. *Atma*, the Soul, is ever free. Otherwise, there can be no search for Reality. Due to ignorance of the Soul, we dwell in the senses. To eliminate this ignorance, the *rishis* discovered various paths to realize the Atma (the Self): the path of knowledge, the path of action, the path of love, and the path of watching and studying the mind. These methods may differ on the starting point, but they lead to the same goal: Self-realization. Krishna, in the Bhagavad Gita, says that knowledge and yoga are one, but the ignorant imagine them to be different.

Jnana Yoga is a path in which the aspirant distinguishes between the real and the unreal by discrimination and by experience. Man is blessed with head, heart, and hands, which are respectively meant for *jnana, bhakti,* and *karma.* Karma cannot be perfect without knowledge and love. Bhakti cannot be understood without action and knowledge. Jnana cannot be gained without love and action. They are all interrelated; true knowledge, true love, and true action can only be acquired by following the path of yoga. Till the body and mind are purged of all impurities by regular practice and adherence to the disciplines of these paths, knowledge cannot be complete, love cannot be full, and action cannot be unselfish. So the yoga of the culture of body and mind is an essential factor in the art of living and realization.

2.2. Health is not something given already complete; it is something to build. You have to build yourselves and create within yourselves the feelings of beauty, liberation, and infinity.

2.3. It is through the body that everything comes to the mind. It is through and with your body that you have to reach realization of being a spark of divinity. How can we neglect the temple of the spirit?

2.4. Before peace between the nations, we have to find peace inside that small nation which is our own being.

2.5. Whatever religion you follow, the body should be sound.

2.6. Everybody should live quietly, whether his experiences are happy or sad, whether they are successes or failures. That is contentment.

2.7. When *kundalini* wakes up, it is very chaotic, and one needs a very strong body to be able to stand it without damaging oneself. We are just like a bulb that bursts if we submit it to an excessive current: this is why training is necessary.

2.8. If the body is in bad health, you cannot expect to find the truth that is in it.

2.9. Freedom is also in our body, the independence of every limb with regard to its neighbor.

2.10. Nothing is perfect; you can always improve. That is creation of life, creation of interest. You must never repeat: a repetition is dead. You must always animate and create interest in whatever you are doing. [*He does the first standing pose.*] This is a perfect asana. Nobody can tell me it has any defect. It is perfect but dead; my mind is elsewhere. Now I shall do it with my mind, I shall create unity within me, and everything will be different.

2.11. In whatever you are doing, be one: body, soul, mind. Do it beautifully and with purity.

2.12. *A Norwegian journalist asked Iyengar: "What is love?"*
Look at Noëlle's feet: those tiny rings were given to her when she arrived in India. Since then she never separated from them. That is love.

2.13. You have suffered a lot in your own body. Now, when someone comes and tells you he is suffering, you feel in your own body what it is to suffer; your personal experience provides you with great love and compassion. So you say: "My friend, let me try and do something."

2.14. It is a wrong approach to be willing to forget this in order to concentrate on that—the mind will escape somewhere else. But if you are one with what you are doing, you forget effort, and unity arises. When a child is playing, is he elsewhere? Go back to childhood.

2.15. Regarding your friend: why should he bother about his experiences? He has to surrender all his experiences to God. Then he will have the harmonious sensation. He should not devote time to certain supernatural experiences that are not the aim of yoga. I have shown you the quotation from Patanjali. He should stick to his method and start the day's work with the Lord's name in his mouth, and surrender everything to Him. He is only an instrument.

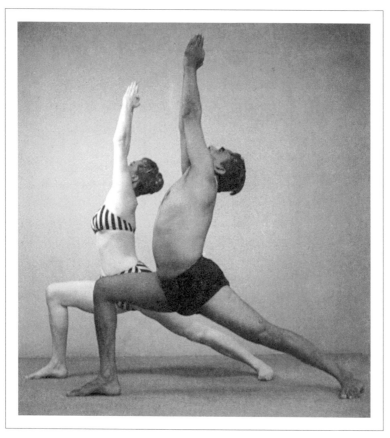

IYENGAR AND NOËLLE IN VIRABHADRASANA I

He should not talk of his feelings apart from surrendering. This also I have shown to you in Patanjali. That may be the final straw if he goes on thinking of his past experiences rather than facing yoga afresh again. I have told you often what suffering and thrilling experiences I underwent, and at the same time even these frightening experiences were bygone things. The only advice

I can give is that your friend should not brood on past experiences, but on the contrary, if it has not done ill in any way, he should calmly pursue his practices as a divine command.

Let him not say, "I have no one who can guide me." I also have no one, yet I depend on the inner command. God remains in the heart of yoga practitioners who are sincere in their efforts. Thus He takes care of them. As he is perfect in other activities, he need not bother much. Only let him start with the name of the Lord and end with the name of the Lord; then he has a balanced approach.

2.16. The lotus grows in muddy waters, but this flower does not show any trace of it. So we have to live in the world.

2.17. Health is a state of complete harmony of body, mind, and spirit, a complete forgetfulness of the physical, resulting in perfect mental peace. When one is free from physical disabilities and mental distractions, the gates to the kingdom of *Atma* (Soul) are opened. The science of yoga deals with both body and mind.

2.18. Philosophy is not an intellectual science, a subject of words and discussion; it's the very art of living.

2.19. We should have a purpose, see it clearly, then get detached from it completely and work.

2.20. Usually when a person has mastered a pose, it becomes uninteresting for him. That is why you can see many people doing mechanically the same thing over and over again, but their mind is elsewhere. It is not the way to approach.

People think they have attained the end. How can they know? It may be only a beginning, or it may be nothing at all. You must always see if you can go further.

2.21. *At the death of N's father*: The spirit is eternal. That cannot die. Your father went to the permanent abode where he came from. Let me pray for his soul to rest in peace. Let his soul bless you to carry on your mission in life. Time is the only healer. Time is the only friend. God will give you strength to bear this heavy loss.

2.22. I have to adjust the expenses of my family according to my earnings; since two months, it is still bad. I have surrendered to the will of God and am peaceful.

2.23. To sit in Lotus Pose and gaze at one's nose is said to be a spiritual practice; to do Lotus Pose and concentrate on the coccyx or elsewhere is said to be a physical practice. Where is the difference? How can Hatha Yoga be only physical and Raja Yoga only spiritual?

2.24. Gross, fine, and infinite: body, mind, and spirit.

2.25. I am really happy that we are together again [in Gstaad]. May God give me strength to help you in your endeavors.

2.26. The yogi, through certain postures, is supposed to be able to eliminate the cobra's poison, death even. It is symbolism: the yogi eliminates toxins, moral and physical impurities, and does not fear death any longer, that's all.

2.27. The *mudra* where the forefinger is joined to the thumb is only a mudra; it has nothing to do with losing energy, as energy could escape through the other fingers, and then we should not cut our nails. It means: "I unite my mind to the Cosmic Mind." So I shall try to meditate. The mudra was done, now it is finished, I can drop it.

2.28. As long as the body is not in perfect health, you think about it, and that prevents you from thinking of the mind. A sound mind in a sound body.

2.29. Without a body, it is impossible to see God. The body has to undergo some training in order to be an effectual help to reach the highest goal: *Atma-darsan* [Self-realization]. For that you need a sound and strong body.

2.30. Find time to do yoga. You should do the asana with vigor and at the same time be relaxed and composed.

2.31. *X hurt one of his toes*: Cut it off and throw it away.

2.32. *Is it necessary to practice all these asana and to push them further and further?*
     Is it necessary to develop scientific researches further and further? To a yogi, the body is a laboratory, a field of experiments and perpetual researches.

2.33. To those who do not believe in God because they do not see Him, I answer: Do you see your back? No? Then does that mean it does not exist? It does exist. Why? Because you retire within yourselves and experience your body. Retire within yourselves and you will find God.

2.34. *A Norwegian journalist asked: "What is the technique of levitation?"*

Iyengar sat down, crossed his legs in Lotus Pose, placed his hands on the floor next to his thighs, and lifted himself. Then he let himself drop the pose heavily, and did it again about four or five times. Then he said: "This is the technique of levitation. There is a quicker and safer way of doing it: it is to love God so much that He draws you up from above."

2.35. Yehudi Menuhin plays music on the violin; it is with his violin that he expresses the Divinity within him. I play yoga asana on my body. What is the difference? How can we say playing on the violin is spiritual work and performance of asana is merely physical?

2.36. If asana demonstrators are judged from the outside, many of them can be called good. To be able to judge the character's value, we have to see if the eyes remain personal or if they become impersonal—which does not mean dead. As long as there is a character (subject) doing asana or actions (objects), there is no divinity, no unity. But when this very character forgets himself completely in his action or asana, he then experiences the Divine and recreates unity.

2.37. *To Queen Elizabeth of Belgium*: "I can't be your teacher and call you Your Majesty. Please, Your Majesty, do this, and so on."

Queen Elizabeth: "Call me Elizabeth."

Iyengar: "No, I will call you Madam."

2.38. *Iyengar told N a story from Narayan Parvan*: For the sake of the world, devils must be killed by a very special sword. For that purpose, the great yogi Dadica was asked to give his spine. He concentrated; then he willingly offered his body. Once his spirit had slipped into the universal conscious-

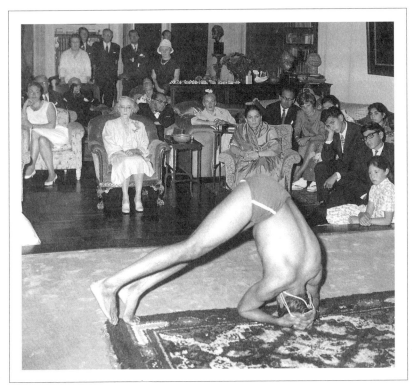

ness, a sword was made out of his bones, and mankind was saved. Iyengar explained to N: "In reality, what are the devils but egoism, jealousy, bad working of the organs, and what are the angels but harmony, love, and balance, etc. Both the good and bad nerves branch out from the spine."

2.39. If we live a negative life, we are inviting discordance between body and mind.

2.40. It is from the spinal column that all the nerves come, and each ends in a pore of the skin. You must control each nerve and each centimeter of the skin.

2.41. When the gardener plants an apple seed, is he enjoying himself thinking of the apples to come? No! He is happy for the first sprouting; he is happy each day for the progress of the plant. Our body is the same. We take care of it by the asana with love and enjoy ourselves seeing the small progress. But we never think of illumination. If it does not come in one year, we work one year more, but without holding fast, otherwise illumination will never come.

2.42. The sleeping tortoise takes all its limbs into its carapace. So does the yogi: going back into himself he does not see anything worldly any longer, he makes peace in himself.

2.43. Man was blessed with a head, a heart, and hands that are made for: *jnana, bhakti,* and *karma.* Karma cannot be done without knowledge and love. Bhakti cannot be understood without action and knowledge. Jnana cannot be gained without love and action. These three are intimately connected. True knowledge, true love, true action cannot be acquired without a regular practice and without adopting rigorous discipline. Otherwise: Knowledge cannot be complete, love cannot be total, action cannot be disinterested.

2.44. K's followers speak a lot about *Atma* (Soul) and feign disinterest for the body, this body we shall soon have to leave. So why was Mr. Y so well dressed? Why were they all eating? Why did they all like to sleep? There is no balance here. All the great sages recommend us to take care of the Temple of the Mind. It should be looked after, fed, provided with all it needs. In this way it will not disturb you any longer and will be a good servant.

We should eat thinking we are getting back some strength in order to serve God. So with all our actions. We should also think that we do not live by ourselves, but that God bears us as the tortoise bears the world in the story of the churning of the milk sea.

The great sages used to say: "How can I put my feet on the ground, I am walking on God."

2.45. When *samadhi* comes, it is as if a 220v current went through a 110v bulb. Either the bulb burns out—that is why it is said that yoga may be dangerous—or one has taken care to transform the bulb. That is why you have to do yoga to strengthen the nervous system.

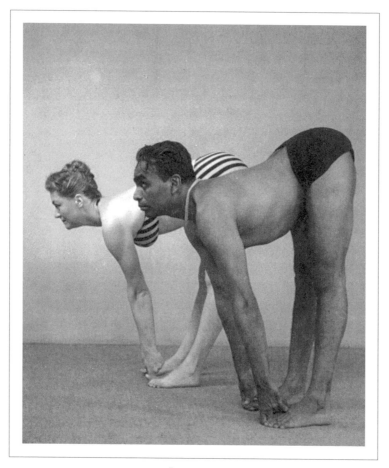

IYENGAR AND NOËLLE IN PADANGUSTHASANA

1961

3.1. Yoga is effort. Only practice is important. The rest of knowledge is only theory.

3.2. It pleases me to hear that your pupils love you and are keen to help you. May you be blessed like that forever through them. I am glad also that they liked my little talks.

3.3. I am sorry to note that you have fewer pupils. All our works are like waves. They go up and down. Last month I started my classes, but I am in the same boat as you. What can I do? I overworked there [in Europe]. I have taken this as God's will and accepted the loss of tuitions here. I may get them back later.

3.4. I agree that financial security is essential. God will take care of you if you have full faith in Him and surrender to Him completely.

3.5. Do the asana thoughtfully with the name of God on the lips.

3.6. Regarding pranayama, the method you wrote is alright. We should learn to devote our practices moment to moment to God. May the name of Jesus remain ever on your lips.

3.7. Be careful with your back, and do the asana thoughtfully, with the name of God on the lips.

3.8. Guruji [Krishnamacharya] was here again and blessed me fully. His blessing will go a long way. He watched my teaching and practice of asana and pranayama. He is impressed beyond measure. He has taught me nothing new, but his blessing will lead me to the right method and a new approach.

3.9. If we face suffering and accept it as a necessary means, all anxiousness disappears.

3.10. My Guruji was here for ten days. Though I spent in all Rs 1,500, it was a great joy for me and my wife to have him in my small house. And I felt that his grace in me was full. He said that he was proud of me and blessed us all. I shall send you sometime later a photo of him taken here, for yourself.

3.11. X will be a fine person beyond what he has been, provided he develops an even mind in all things at all times. May God bless him; for me I am not God. I have my human weakness and try to improve.

Please convey my love to Koko; whatever he thinks of me of late will do no justice to him. I am as I was and ever will be. I know only to work with interest and with honesty; the rest of Tantra Yoga is not for me. My yoga is a different one: to work and surrender to the Lord.

3.12. The world is full of people who say that only they are right and their system is the best. Nobody thinks or acts without making a choice. Yoga is not as bad as people think. What hurts me more is people giving opinions on subjects which are unknown to them. That shakes the layman. But it is common, and one has to laugh when people speak on a subject unknown to them.

3.13. I got a little money in Europe, and God wants me to remain content even if I do not make much here. I surrender to His wishes and live happily.

3.14. Never go to an asana with aggressiveness.

3.15. Go quickly to your maximum; then only use your energy to improve.

3.16. As we shave, it happens that we cut ourselves with the razor blade; this does not mean that we must not shave in the morning any longer. It is the same thing for yoga.

3.17. Do the asana without fail but not aggressively; get control on all, but without strain. Do your work well, and feel moment to moment as though it is the service you are doing for the Lord. Do think of Him.

3.18. Only patience pays. One has to persevere.

3.19. I have also increased the intensity in asana and find new things in each asana. It is a joy to do them, watching the changes.

3.20. Next year, if things go well, we will meet again. Whatever time is possible for me to spare in my busy program, please accept with joy. I appreciate you and your efforts, so do not lose heart. God will bless you.

3.21. I am happy that all in my house are yoga and music conscious. Now God has only to give these children the mind to persist in their knowledge.

3.22. Do pranayama as dedication to Lord Christ. It is pranayama and prayer combined. To do it is good.

3.23. I hope you are recovering from all your weaknesses. These things are to be sustained, and we should maintain and remain calm and proceed in the aim that is our goal.

3.24. I hope that you will improve with your pains and be a happy woman again. You have taken a hard path like me. Suffering has become a mainstay with me and with you.

1962

4.1. Meditation is when you are one with yourself. If a woman who is cooking is completely absorbed by her cooking, it is meditation. You never know when meditation is going to happen; it falls upon you, it rapes you. You cannot say, I am going to meditate. Meditation is not the work of unification; it is oneness. It is only later on that we become aware it happened in a split second, although time does not exist in meditation (not unification, but oneness).

4.2. May God bless you, your friends, and your pupils with long life, happiness, and peace within.

4.3. I am patiently doing all with aches and pains. I make good progress, and again I fall back. Nowadays I do so many things, and the next day I am out. Yet with strong will I pursue my efforts as though they are the commands of God. My knee pain and hip pain have remained. The knee is better now, but the catch in the hip does not go. It comes while I am teaching due to the support I give, keeping my body in different positions. There is a gentleman who comes to the class. He is so big that when he sits on a chair, his abdo-

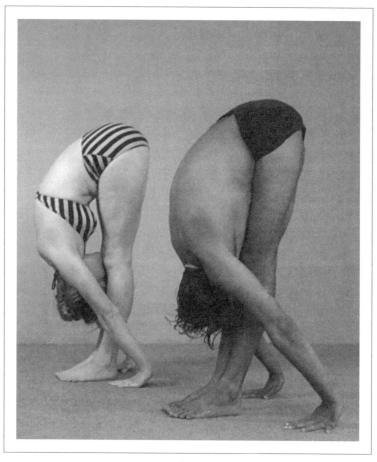

IYENGAR AND NOËLLE IN UTTANASANA

men touches his knees. So big, so huge, he needs several bulldozers to lift him. I have to work with my two bare hands.

4.4. Do not worry about this person saying he has seen his own image in his spleen. One has to see oneself through one's actions, works, and mind. Knowing the Self by the self is not as easy as writing that line. A yogi sees things in every movement he makes, maybe when practicing, maybe when teaching, or maybe when talking to people. You should have courage in your convictions and pursue what is dear to you all these years.

4.5. We must absorb everything without a conditioned mind. Fear and tiredness condition the mind to say no, although the body could do it. All this stands against the work.

4.6. Sometimes everything within us objects so much to work and we doubt so strongly that in order not to give up we have to find a means to work at all costs.

4.7. To master fear is the most important battle to win.

4.8. Like a snake, the spine should move from end to end; when the head moves, the movement is transmitted up to the tail.

4.9. Your mind is already well ahead of your body. So you have to conquer the pains of the body and get harmony and cooperation.

4.10. Regarding your pupil, Mr. X, he has to trust you and do it. He cannot get anywhere by jumping from teacher to teacher. For me, the way he follows comes from a doubtful mind. Nothing can be achieved with a mind that doubts others.

4.11. It is necessary to practice with faith, patience, and persistence. It is not a question of "do yoga and feel fine." It has to be worked deeply. After thirty years of practice, I now do the asana with comfort and ease.

4.12. Intelligence alone does not solve anything. First, observation is necessary, then one can use the brain.

4.13. N: *"This A is wonderful. When you show him something, he does it at once."*

"That is called frustration, Madam. It is the difference between your approach and mine. You want to do a pose to master it and put it in your pocket; I do it to do it. Be detached from the results."

4.14. In yoga, three very important things have always to be united in everything: love, knowledge, and action.

4.15. *Sadhana* should be pursued even though pain and death are at our throat.

4.16. Though things go to pieces for you, remain in peace.

4.17. God is kind to me in every way. Only I have to strain more than my capacity. It is something that must be borne so that God's will can be carried out.

1963

5.1. Love must be incarnated in the smallest pore of the skin, the smallest cell of the body, to make them intelligent, so they can collaborate with all the other ones, in the big republic of the body.

5.2. Things have to take their own shape. I leave it to God.

5.3. I am sorry to know that you are not getting students. Hope members will arrive soon. Do not get disheartened. It is a test of the Lord. Face it calmly. He will come to your help.

5.4. Relaxation means emptiness.

5.5. The eyes must go to the region that does not work, not to the one that does.

5.6. From head to heels, find your center.

5.7. The goal of yoga is known. If we fail to reach it, soon we feel darkness everywhere. We have to gain confidence and face these trials.

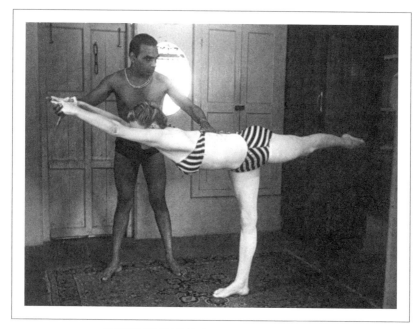

IYENGAR WITH NOËLLE IN VIRABHADRASANA III

5.8. Problems will exist up to the end of your life. It is not a reason to drop the practice of yoga.

5.9. Do not worry about small things. He has his own way of measuring men and matters; others have their own way. Do not bother about it. When he meets you again, you can ask him to forget the incident. If he still sticks to his views, you can forget about it. That is the yoga way of mental peace. Do not bother about that past incident with B. Better think of God and your pupils.

5.10. I don't know how the pains have not left you. I hope God's grace falls on you soon and you are relieved of these ugly patches in your life.

5.11. While doing the postures, your mind should be in half-consciousness, which does not mean sleep. It means silence, emptiness, space, which can then be filled with an acute awareness of the sensations given by the posture. You watch yourself from inside. It is a full silence.

5.12. The body has to be invaded by the intelligence; each part has to become intelligent.

5.13. When the active brain becomes passive, the passive brain becomes active. That is meditation. Meditation is unknown to you; a known is not meditation, because the known comes as an object and hinders the subject to be in the subject.

5.14. Communion is union. Observe, when you do asana, if the body is active, if the brain is active. When both are active it is called yoga; it is communion, it is union.

5.15. *Gu* = light. *Ru* = ignorance. He who removes ignorance is a Guru. The Guru is a man who drives you from darkness to light.

5.16. You must be as joyful when you fail again and again as you are joyful when you succeed. It is often when you fail that you move toward the goal without being aware of it. You must feel joy even when you have not fully succeeded but only moved toward achievement of your goal.

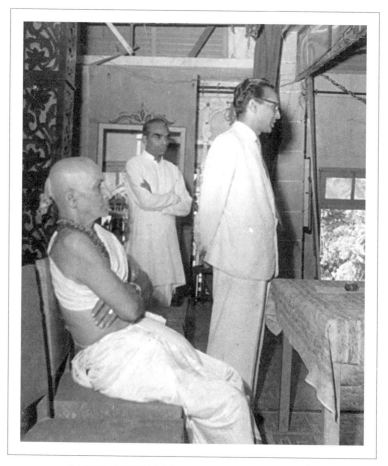

T. KRISHNAMACHARYA AND B.K.S IYENGAR, PUNE, 1961

1964

6.1. Passivity while working comes afterward, when the posture is perfect; before that a tremendous effort is required. At your level, effort comes first. At my level, what comes first is zeal; there are almost no painful efforts.

6.2. *There was a gadfly resting on Iyengar, so I asked him, "Can I kill it?"*
"Oh, yes," he said.
I killed it and added laughingly, "See how bad a Brahmin you are!"
He laughed and answered, "You did not read the Manusmriti. There he says that killing to protect others is not bad. Manu was the first to write on Hindu laws; he wrote that we can kill harmful beasts. He was living around the Christian era. I like to translate *ahimsa* as 'not to harm' rather than 'not to kill.'"

6.3. I am sorry to note that you lost your dear grandmother. Last time I missed paying my respects to her. May her soul rest in peace. Joys and sorrows go together, only at times we feel we are mostly in sorrow.

6.4. I hope you have a fine time now in Paris, and I wish you a bright future and good financial success through yoga teaching, and spiritual joy through yoga practice.

6.5. All of you are attached to your body; you are afraid, so you protect yourself. Be detached. Look at me, I am not afraid, and I do not spare myself any difficulties. You Westerners are attached to the body, and you always want to improve. For me, if it came yesterday, so much the better; if it comes only after twenty years, so much the better. All is well; do not be attached.

6.6. In one of the Upanishads, a young man goes and asks a wise man to become his Guru and to teach him the path of realization (nonduality). The Guru agrees, provided that the man takes his cow and comes back one day with a herd of 1,000 cows. He agrees. Then one day at last the 1,000 cows are there, so he goes back to his Guru, who asks him what he did during all this time. He answered that his only occupation had been to develop his herd as quickly as possible. So the Guru said, "You know the way, I have got nothing more to teach you."

6.7. A young man goes to meet a wise man, asking him to become his Guru. The Guru gives him a pot of milk and asks him to carry it on his head and walk without losing a single drop of milk. The man places the pot on his head, follows the circuit, and comes back.

The Guru asks him, "How many women did you meet?"

"I do not know."

"Did you meet the king's son?"

"I do not know."

"So, what did you do?"

"I walked, trying not to lose a single drop of milk."

"Then," the Guru said, "you do not need me. You know the way already."

6.8. Patanjali doesn't say that yoga is union, but concentration.

6.9. I am as busy as I was. It is physical and mental strain, too. Though I am working hard, I am not free from pains and sorrows. Being a teacher, I have to swallow my pains. My body is already broken while teaching, and there is no more room for further cracks. I used to tell you, kicks and bumps brought out all my teeth. Now you also have started experiencing the same. That is our true selfless *sadhana*. For the good of others, we suffer.

6.10. In my book, I wrote about standing poses, legs three feet or five feet apart, according to the postures. But to be contented with that is meaningless. According to what we want to work, we must spread the legs more or less.

6.11. *Here is a* sloka *Iyengar sang in Sanskrit to help us hold a pose*: Old ladies speak of chastity and control because their glands do not work any longer.

6.12. Complete self-oblivion: The only way I can explain it is by analogy with sexual enjoyment. Although one is animal and sensuous while the other is reached through yoga, in both cases self-oblivion is total.

6.13. *Buddhi* = wisdom: the wisdom that comes by work, the knowledge that comes by experience.

6.14. Hard work and genius bring talent.

6.15. God is great. Nehru has gone. His ideals will never leave us. We have great men, but they may not come to the height of Mr. Nehru. We have lost Gandhi, now Nehru. They are the leaders of humanity. God save us.

6.16. Take care while teaching not to strain your back. While teaching you may not feel it, but later you may suffer. As you say that you have less work, take it as a blessing from the Lord for the time being. Take things as they come, peacefully.

6.17. God is one; it is the sages who gave Him different names.
   The other day, he said: Alberto is not a God, but God's name is Alberto.

6.18. Suicide is not an answer; it is mental imbalance. She has to surrender to God and do what you teach her faithfully. Without faith, she will not go ahead much.

6.19. The seat of the Lord, some people say, is situated in the heart, others say in the head. They try to concentrate there and believe they are meditating. In fact they do nothing. It is mere emptiness, and they are not present everywhere. However, if you prick your finger, or if a mosquito bites you, you react, which means that the Mind, Life, Being are present there, too.

Take a wheel; is it made only of the nave? No, it is also made of the spokes and the rim. We have to go constantly from the nave to the rim and from the rim to the nave through the spokes. It is the same for the human being: it is only then that we are present to life. The seat of Life is everywhere. Do not think that you are with God or that you are meditating because you are sitting with closed eyes and trying hopelessly to go down to a so-called seat of Life.

6.20. I want awareness in awareness; only that is creation.

6.21. If you speak of a nice feeling or of a perfect balance, you ruin this same feeling, which is completely alive and which is already a moment of eternity.

6.22. During the times of the great *rishis*, everybody was religious, the world walked on the four legs of religion. However, it used to be said that many penances were required to see God. Now you are told to go and see a guru who will give you a vision of God, without you making any effort. All this is a lie, and it is done to cheat credulous people.

6.23. Realization is oneness and not unification. It is unity, dissolved duality, fusion, nonduality.

6.24. In India, 90 percent of love marriages do not last; it is not love but desire.

6.25. Yoga is also called by Patanjali *yoga-darsana,* or "mirror," because we look at ourselves from inside to see what is working and what is not working. Controlling the mind is yoga. When the mind is controlled, what remains? The soul. It is the very purpose of yoga.

6.26. You must go from the known to the unknown and come back to the known. It is impossible to say, I am going to meditate, or I meditated for two hours. If we know it lasted two hours, we were in the self and not in the Infinite, where there is no more time.

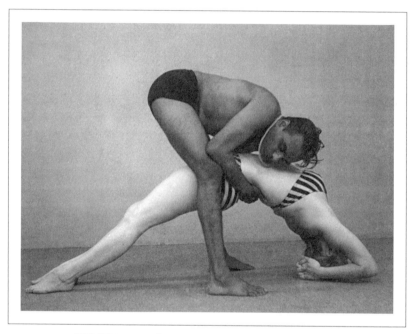

IYENGAR WITH NOËLLE IN DWI PADA VIPARITA DANDASANA

1965

7.1. Intelligence has to penetrate the muscles and enable us to execute the asana perfectly. We reach the Self only through the conquest of all parts of the body.

7.2. I came to teach you how to face despair.

7.3. *Iyengar:* "Yoga begins only when *kundalini* is awakened. What you do before is only the foundation. Kundalini is a beginning, not an end, as many people believe."

    A: "If kundalini is the beginning, what is the end?"

    Iyengar laughed. "Who knows?"

7.4. As a sculptor should express God (Being, perfection, beauty) through stone, bronze or wood, I should express God through my whole being, my thoughts, my soul, my body, my love.

7.5. North is the top of the head,
    East is the front,

West is the back,
South, the feet.

7.6. *Iyengar shows A the difference between my left side and my right, and goes on:* Everyone has a side which is better than the other. Balance between *Ha*, the right, and *Tha*, the left, is yoga. Perfect harmony means perfect control and a deep research; that is yoga.

7.7. Regarding X, I have to see again. Do carefully, watchfully, and thoughtfully; you may discover the defect and find the way for relief.

7.8. I planted the seed, now you must work a lot, otherwise the tiny plant will die.

7.9. To do something for the results is greed. When a pupil arrives, he has a small purpose. While working he loses it, as he discovers that he can go much further; then he is pure. If he catches a second purpose, again he is not pure; he has to lose it again.

7.10. I am glad to know that you do not have heavy pupils. I hope this continues for a long time, so that you gain strength. You have also overdone, and your body needs rest. It is a blessing of God that you have fewer pupils. Maybe soon, God may provide you more. For that He is giving you rest to gain strength.

7.11. Silence in silence is the beginning of meditation. But before you have this experience you can't understand, so I don't explain it to you.

7.12. *In Trikonasana, touching A's head he said,* "There is Brahma; there is Siva." Then, touching the buttocks, "There is Sakti."

"Purusa?" asked A.

"Yes, Purusa means consciousness. In the head is the passive brain, here the active brain. Sakti has to move and be Siva; then it is meditation. But you want to act with the head and you forget the buttocks. That is a contradiction: you make passive what has to be active and active what has to be passive, so that *kundalini* cannot go into *susumna* without hindrance."

7.13. When I ask you to stretch your spine, you stretch in the middle where *susumna* is, but you should relax in the middle and stretch on both sides. *Sakti* will be free only then.

7.14. Meditation is really to do everything with love, not to sit and close the eyes and utter the name of God mechanically. That is a waste of time.

7.15. More than twenty years ago, I told Krishnaji that a frustrated being cannot find God.

7.16. When you come, you have frames in your mind; you think. As soon as your hand opens my door, you lose your frames of mind, ready to follow my instructions. Then while working, you escape again into your thoughts, so I shout, "I want this," and you are frightened, and your mind is again freed of its frames. At that very moment, it is pure morality, what you call virtue.

7.17. Do your postures carefully, with understanding. Do not miss doing yoga, but do it thoughtfully. May God bless you.

Do yoga carefully, watchfully, and thoughtfully. You may find the defect and find the way for relief.

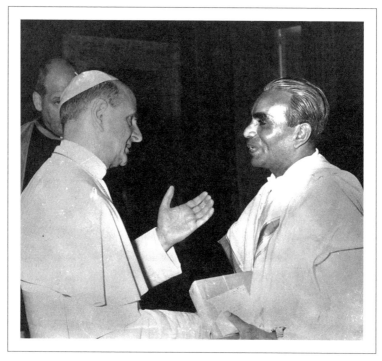

IYENGAR WITH HIS HOLINESS POPE PAUL VI, ROME, 1966

7.18. Service to humanity is service to God, and the means for that is yoga.

7.19. Space brings precision. Precision brings freedom. Freedom brings truth (*satya*). Truth is God.

1966

8.1. People may speak of truth and the essence of life, but inside they are jealous, selfish, and like to save their skin.

8.2. How can I lose my temper if you do not correspond with me? After all, we think of each other. A day may not pass without us thinking of each other.

8.3. *From Italy.* Here I met His Holiness the Pope on the 27th at 12 noon. He was very happy to have met me and praised my book, my work, and blessed me several times. We were together for eight minutes, and during that time he was holding my arms firmly and spoke of India and Indians and the affection he has towards my country. He said, "As you are a professor and a director, what more have I to tell you, when you have done such wonderful work." The audience was at Castel Gandolfo. It was a memorable moment. He is a very nice man, sweet in heart.

This year, when things were not at all going in my favor, this meeting with the Pope was the greatest event of the year. He presented me with a medal as a souvenir of our meeting. I was in my Indian *dhoti* and shawl. I presented him with a sandalwood walking stick. He touched it, felt it, smelled it, and said, "Very fine." I asked to give a demonstration of yoga, but he said he was very busy. I asked him twice to grant me permission. He said that he loves yoga but has no time now, as he is very busy. He blessed me several times and wished me well in my field.

8.4. *About Scorpion Pose*: The yogi, by stamping on his head with his feet, attempts to eradicate the self-destroying emotions and passions. By kicking his head, he seeks to develop humility, calmness, and tolerance and thus be free of ego. The subjugation of ego leads to harmony and happiness.

1967

9.1. If art goes according to the whims of a particular person, there is no more Truth.

9.2. People do not act for their own sake, but to please another, which is irreligious.

9.3. The capital we are born with, the human body, lies unutilized for the great majority of us.

9.4. For yogis who go out of their way to help those who come, fatigue is our nature. It is the birthright of a yoga teacher. So we have to accept the fatigue and work with intense awareness to gain back energy. Awareness in action brings back a lot of energy.

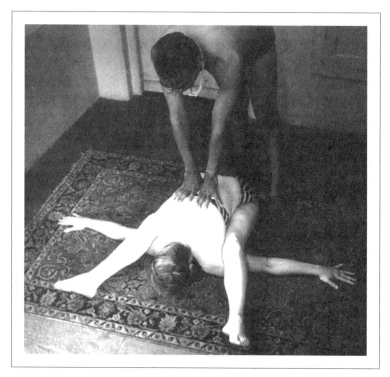

IYENGAR WITH NOËLLE IN KURMASANA

1968

10.1. If I come this year, I hope we can meet at least once and speak for a day or two about ourselves, our progress, and our experiences.

10.2. Throw a hint, nothing happens. Throw a hit, and see what happens!

10.3. It is never a question of what I am doing but what am I not doing.

10.4. You must develop the same character as the *kurma*, the tortoise. When once it is in its shell, nothing at all can disturb it. In Kurmasana, you are unable to see anyone or anything, obliging you to turn your attention inwards.

10.5. How happy I am to hear from you. We are all in the same boat. Life is hard. I am also working as hard as before. No peace for people like us. It is we who shouldered it, so we have to accept this type of life.

10.6. A battle ensues when the mind says, "I want to," but the body says, "I can't." It is in one's own hands to see who wins.

10.7. The end of discrimination is the beginning of wisdom. Discrimination means that doubt is still there. When doubt has completely gone, there will be no need of discrimination.

10.8. Life is very hard in India, as in Paris. We work more as we grow older to make both ends meet. Life is hard. Yet one has to continue.

10.9. I am glad that you are having a very busy time and it is leading you to forget your very existence. That is a good sign, because you live in divinity while you are engaged in teaching.

10.10. You cannot say you are intelligent if you do not also have body intelligence.

10.11. The body is an institution. The teacher is within.

10.12. The East is truly a spiritual country. She has sent jewels out into the West, and always they have drawn thousands of Westerners into their radiance. India is not a passive, useless country. She is still performing her miracles in this way in teaching humanity in the wider world, spreading her message beyond Indian shores.

10.13. The yogic pranayama, or breathing techniques, are meditative in their origin and in their effect. Consisting basically of breath inhalation, breath retention, and breath exhalation, their rhythmic movement stills the mind by withdrawing the senses and helps one uncover the depths of the Self.

10.14. Memory is useless if it brings about a repetition of the past. Memory is useful if it helps to prepare you for the future, to know whether or not you are proceeding forward.

10.15. Giving does not impoverish, nor does withholding enrich us.

10.16. *With regard to Surya Namaskar*: We are always seeking contact with Heaven. But how many of us have made any reasonable contact with Mother Earth?

10.17. Westerners are certainly intellectually more developed than the average Easterner, but emotionally more immature. Westerners tend to rationalize or brood over things, over what they can do to get over or change their pain, which is an escape from actually facing it. They are seldom prepared to face that pain and work through it. Take, for example, the terrible shouts, cries, and groans when you are taken intensely into a posture, thus bringing you face to face with the reality of your body's nature. Take also the emotional breakdown in sensitivity training, when you are unavoidably with the reality of your own nature. We must face up to our emotions, not run away from them.

10.18. Sleep is a sensual activity.

10.19. When the means are good, the end cannot but be likewise good. The means must be good, or the end will be meaningless.

10.20. Yoga is nothing if it is not perfect harmony.

10.21. May God bless you forever. May He be a light to you.

10.22. The body is made up of five layers: the anatomical layer, the physiological layer, the psychological layer, the intellectual layer, bliss. Hatha Yoga develops all five layers, not as in Western disciplines, for instance, merely the physiological layer.

10.23. A teacher must first have demonstrated and experienced in his own life what he is teaching before teaching others.

10.24. The trouble today is that not only are the pupils undisciplined, but their teachers too are similarly undisciplined.

10.25. To know oneself is to know one's body, soul, and mind.

10.26. Any dull posture must be made active.

10.27. Yoga is an art. Yoga is my art.

10.28. People who work very hard and don't get proper nourishment will suffer from low blood pressure.

10.29. Anything that disturbs your spiritual life and practice is a disease.

10.30. The highest form of sensitivity is the highest form of intellect. Where does need end and greed begin? One who knows this has a religious mind.

10.31. Just like a river, the Self has two banks—a material bank and a spiritual bank. *Sadhana* is the boat that takes you from the material to the spiritual bank.

10.32. Purity is when there is no anxiety, no worry, no thinking.

10.33. Morality begins in us.

10.34. Without health, one cannot have a strong root in the mind. The movements of the mind—laziness, carelessness, believing illusion to be the truth—have to be still in order to know what the soul is.

10.35. The end of discipline is the beginning of freedom. Only a disciplined person is a free person. So-called freedom is only a license to act and do as we like. Yoga is meant to train and discipline the worries and anxieties of men and women.

10.36. Freedom in a posture is when every joint is active. Let us be full in whatever posture it is we are doing. Let us be full in whatever we do.

10.37. Life is immortal; death is mortal.

10.38. In your discipline, if doubt comes, let it come. You do your work and let doubt carry on with its work. And let us see which gives up first!

10.39. I live in the body, not in Mauritius, London, India, or South Africa.

10.40. In yoga, the body disciplines the mind and the mind disciplines the body. The mind cannot think of the soul as long as it is connected to the body. The body must be trained to be the servant, not the master.

10.41. Singularity of purpose should be your aim.

10.42. Meditation is a fine, supreme consciousness in which there is no duality.

10.43. The body has to be transformed. It must be brought to stability.

10.44. The body is still in one piece, which is why you are in pieces. The body must be broken down into pieces for there to be peace.

10.45. Health is that state in which one can forget about the body.

10.46. Just as a goldsmith purifies gold, so must the body be constantly purified and purged, so that the inner gold may shine.

10.47. Your skin is a most sensitive guide.

10.48. The mind, the thinker, must be made utterly and completely still to know what the Self is.

10.49. All discipline must come from within. All fire and purity must come from within.

10.50. Nobody should become a graduate if he is unfit in his body. Of what use is a degree if the body is not going to last, if the body is one day going to corrupt that knowledge?

10.51. Through the emotional center, one cultivates the intellect of the heart. Through the intellectual center, one cultivates the intellect of the head.

10.52. The presence or absence of intelligence is shown when you face insecurity. Security lies in insecurity.

10.53. Why think of *moksha,* liberation, at some future time? Liberation is in the little things here and now.

10.54. *At a public lecture*: My dear friends, please do not smoke; you have come to see yoga, not to smoke.

10.55. Man believes that spiritual contact is painful and should be rendered as painless and as brief as possible. Yet, if a journey to outer space demands rigorous discipline covering a period of years, it should be clear that a trip to the transcendent is not that easy.

10.56. The pranayamic techniques, like the asana, are vehicles of meditation and prayers. Breath inhalation, or *puraka,* is acceptance of the Lord. Breath retention, or *kumbhaka* (from a pot filled to the brim with water which is thereafter silent), is savoring of the Lord in the full, deep stillness of the heart. Exhalation, or *recaka,* is not simply exhalation, but it is the emptying of the ego. Exhalation makes one impersonal and hence a fit instrument of surrender to the Lord. It is the highest form of surrender to the Lord.

10.57. It has been maintained that yogic meditation is without content, a mere emptying of the mind. For those who have had the experience of its richness and satisfying fullness, such as assertion can only sound ridiculous. The intellect of the mind may cease its roving, but the intellect of the heart goes out to the Lord. And it is the heart that matters. Is there really need of the petty content of our own thoughts, when the heart is drawn to the Infinite One, who is always near and ever receding, immanent and transcendent at the same time?

10.58. The mind is drawn to surrender to the Holy One. This surrender, by breaking the chain of distracting thoughts, increases the intensity of one's concentration.

10.59. Meditation does not make the mind dull. Rather, in meditation the mind is still but razor sharp, silent but vibrant with energy. But this state cannot be achieved without a firm, stable sitting posture, where the spine ascends and the mind descends and dissolves in the consciousness of the heart, where the true Self reveals itself.

10.60. The mind integrates the body and yet remains an observer; the body becomes mind and yet remains supremely alert as body. And so mind and matter are fused in the dynamism of sheer energy, which is active without being spent, creative without bringing on exhaustion.

10.61. The whole body, far from being ignored, is taken up in this spiritual alertness, till the whole man becomes pure flame. An alert, erect spine creates a spiritual intensity of concentration that burns out distracting thoughts and the brooding over past and future, and leaves one in the virginal, fresh present.

10.62. Why develop like a racehorse, as it is the case with so many wrestlers, athletes, and gymnasts? In the course of time, the racehorse becomes a carthorse.

10.63. Generally, in India, those who practice yoga do it for the culmination of births. But I say that one should not bother about having more life, as it gives more chances for man to think of God. If it is God's will, let him give me a thousand lives, but let him leave his name to be on my tongue forever.

10.64. It is the job of the spine to keep the brain alert and in position.

10.65. God requires only this of us: that we learn to distinguish between that which is spiritual and that which is sensual.

10.66. God is our pupils. We need not seek God elsewhere. So devote yourself to this art, which is a vehicle to see God through the people whom He sends us.

10.67. The intellect needs to be humbled for the body to become the temple of God.

10.68. Irritability is a measure of insanity. If the pupil becomes irritable, the teacher must treat him likewise with irritability.

10.69. If a man has valor but his sword is rusty, of what use is his valor? If a man has spiritual aspirations but his body is corrupt, of what use are his aspirations?

10.70. If you look after the root of the tree, the fragrance and flowering of the tree will come of itself. If you look after the body, the fragrance of the mind and spirit will come of itself.

10.71. During a posture, suffer now, cry later.

10.72. In India, in ancient times, everyone, no matter what path of yoga was chosen, had to undergo asana-pranayama training.

10.73. Yoga aims for complete awareness in everything you do.

10.74. What is the use of merely developing the muscles, if the brain is not working?

10.75. Anything that sustains and supports is religious. If you are well and allow yourself to become unwell, that is being irreligious. To lift up someone who is about to fall or who has fallen is religious.

10.76. The spine brings physical stability, the mind brings emotional stability, the brain brings intellectual stability.

10.77. A crooked body means a crooked mind. It's a crooked mind that says, "I think I can." Be positive! Never say, "I'm trying." If you were trying, you wouldn't be able to open your mouth to say anything.

10.78. Too much eating, talking, and walking must be stopped.

10.79. Most Westerners try to solve their emotional problems through the intellect of the head. Emotions can, however, only be solved through the emotions.

10.80. Yoga works not with the physical body but with the physiological body.

10.81. In ancient times, pupils went in search of gurus. Today gurus go in search of pupils. That's why spirituality has lost its fragrance.

10.82. Analytical intelligence is easy to acquire, but not practical intelligence.

10.83. You have to work through the gross body to the subtle body (the spine), and then through the spine to the mind.

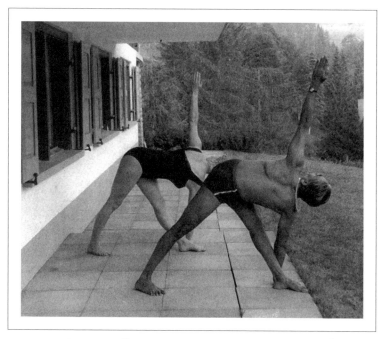

IYENGAR AND NOËLLE IN PARIVRTTA TRIKONASANA, GSTAAD, 1965

1969

11.1. It is very difficult to synthesize everything and to draw out the common center that is good for everyone.

11.2. In the beginning, I am violent because the body does not know what to do and the mind does not want to follow.

11.3. All people have different constitutions. Never compare. Only compare when there is a good climate between those who are doing the poses.

11.4. Correct from the root.

11.5. Being a family man myself, I well understand how hard it is for us to survive without work and still harder to save for our own protection when in need. We are not saints or *sannyasin* to command help from society. With the same knowledge you or I have, if we were in saffron robes, society would have paid more respect. But that would not have been a true approach for us. Let God bless us so that this hard work assures our maintenance.

11.6. Be so silent that you hear the sound within. Not even the ticking of the clock should disturb you.

11.7. My mind is with you when I am in Gstaad. Our work comes to my mind very often. God is very near, yet far. We both are near, yet far. Only my good wishes are always near you.

11.8. May God bless you. My good wishes for you are always there, whether we meet or not. Trust in Him and do your best.

11.9. Detail and precision of the body lead to mastering the art of relaxation.

11.10. To keep the mouth open is going against the will of God. There is a heavy load on the lungs if the mouth is open, and people with heart trouble get pain.

11.11. From concrete meditation go to abstract meditation.

11.12. You should remember always this sentence from the Gita: Lord Krishna says, "To those who worship me alone with single-minded devotion, who are in harmony with me every moment, I bring total security. I shall supply all their wants and shall protect them forever."

11.13. Know your capacity. Each one's capacity is a function of his or her own internal strength.

11.14. You should work to obtain a perfect balance between both sides of the body.

11.15. First you start with physical action; then you have to forget about action on that plane only. You have to discipline the mind through the action.

11.16. Even if intellectually you understand how to reach meditation, in reality, if you do not control your emotions, you will never reach it.

11.17. It is not a loss if you cannot come to Gstaad. After all, you have taken much yoga training from outside you, and now the light has to illuminate from within by your own *sadhana*. May that light shine on you.

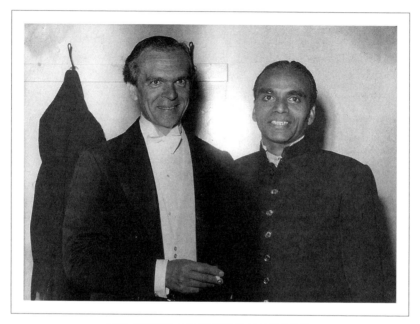

B.K.S. IYENGAR AND PIANIST W. MALCUZYNSKI

1970

12.1. Did you come to watch your clock or to do yoga?

12.2. You always have to watch your median line.

12.3. The guru helps the *chela* (pupil) to master fear.

12.4. No pain, no gain in life. This one should know. Nothing comes with ease. If any have that notion, they are wrong.

12.5. Every day, head and neck balance, with the brain completely relaxed. This is far superior to sleep and rest.

12.6. You must have an inquisitive spirit: "Why am I doing this? Why does it happen?"

12.7. The pupil must push the teacher to tears; that is the way to make a good teacher.

12.8. Yoga is the knowledge of the Self. Knowledge of the Self does not imply negligence or carelessness concerning the body and the mind. Knowledge of the Self encompasses knowledge relating to the gross and subtle sheaths of the Self, which have to be purified and perfected by devoted, uninterrupted practice.

12.9. But yoga is all this and more. It makes the sincere practitioner an integrated personality. It helps the harmonious development of body and mind. It develops a feeling of oneness between man and nature, between man and man, and between man and his Maker, thus aiding a feeling of identity with the spirit pervading all creation.

12.10. The ordinary man can be made to understand what yoga is by exploring the concrete—that is, the body. There exists a communion and proper understanding between body and nerves, nerves and mind, mind and intellect, intellect and will, will and consciousness.

When these vehicles of the *jivatma* operate at their highest level of efficiency, then pure awareness alone remains. It is hard to begin directly with the abstract—the Soul—which is *sat-chit-ananda* (existence, consciousness, bliss).

12.11. Yoga is the process of stilling the mind and then merging the individual soul (*jivatma*) with Universal Soul (*Paramatma*).

12.12. Think light! Try to impart a feeling of lightness to the body. Think light. This can be achieved by mentally extending yourself outwards from the center of the body, i.e., think tall. Think not just of raising your arms but of extending them outwards, and when you are holding them still, think again of reaching still farther away from your body. Do not think of yourself as a small, compressed, suffering thing. Think of yourself as graceful and expanding, no matter how unlikely it may seem at the time.

12.13. If God exists, He exists in all of you as laziness.

12.14. *In the car, when I took Iyengar to the airport, he went on:* "After Sarvangasana, if your neck is paining . . ." At Cointrin airport, taking a last cup of coffee: "All emotional troubles, Setu Bandha Sarvangasana on a chair, the emotional center should be more active . . ." After a big farewell, marks of affection for Mummy, another recommendation: "Be careful with yourself, do it for me . . ." Then he came back to the gate and called to me from afar: "When the brain is perfectly calm, then meditation begins."

12.15. You need discipline. To go on with the pose requires endurance. Also, stretch a little bit more. If there is a stretch somewhere that is positive, softness is negative. We must watch and make positive the negative side, and vice versa.

12.16. A confused mind finds a confused teacher.

12.17. When the body is moving, the spine should not be hard; and when the spine is moving, the body has to move with the spine but not be hard. Be attentive.

12.18. When you see a mistake in somebody else, try to find if you are doing the same mistake.

12.19. When one side is more active than the other, the active side must become the guru for the inactive side to make it active. For the weakest side, we must use more intelligence, we must show more care. As we show keener interest and attention to improve a dull, sleepy friend than for an eager, intelligent one, in the same way you have to act on either side of the body.

12.20. If you do not know the silence of the body, you do not know the silence of the mind. Action and silence must go together. Where there is action, there is silence, and where there is silence, there is action.

12.21. I am testing people by asking them to do what they are reluctant to do, and I see whether they persevere or not. So I can also see whether they are sincere.

1971

13.1. God is so near and yet so far.

13.2. What is pain if it enables you to see God?

13.3. Harmony will come only by observation.

13.4. During inhalation, the breath should move exactly like clouds spreading in the sky.

13.5. I hinder nobody from smoking. People smoke because they are unhappy. When they have practiced enough yoga, they become happy and stop smoking by themselves.

13.6. Do not observe from your physical eyes but from the conscious mind, which is a visual mind.

13.7. It is only when you can complete the pose and be relaxed that you can become one with your mind and intellect.

13.8. The moment the body collapses, the brain collapses.

13.9. In spiritual quietness, everything is quiet, even attention.

13.10. There are three types of pupils: the baby monkey, the baby cat, the little fish. The baby monkey clings always to its mother's back. This type of pupil is always dependent on the teacher. The kitten is always restless and runs away, so that his mother must constantly chase him and bring him back. This type of pupil must always be chased after and caught by the master. The little fish, his eyes never close! This pupil is constantly observing and learning.

13.11. Pupils must have a million eyes.

13.12. When the breath is nicely exhaled towards the heart, the heart is purified from the desires and emotions that disturb it.

13.13. The best sign of a good Savasana is a feeling of deep peace and pure bliss. Savasana is a watchful surrendering of the ego. Forgetting oneself, one discovers oneself.

13.14. Without a body, we cannot see God. We are incarnated. We train the body to make it a fit instrument to reach the highest goal, to contemplate Being. To do this, your body must be healthy and strong.

13.15. Balance is a gift of the Creator.

13.16. In whatever position (or condition), one has to find balance.

13.17. Sensory stillness is a state of emptiness and not a state of fullness.

13.18. Yoga is the art of getting rid of borders. Do not cut yourself off from the Infinite with too narrow ideas. Leave always the possibility of saying, "I shall try," "I shall see." Create in the Infinite. Do not be limited beings.

13.19. There is physical need and mental desire. Physical need can be stopped by asana like Virasana, Baddha Konasana, and so on. When sexual desire springs from the mind, it can be stopped by pranayama.

13.20. To know the mind, we have to go beyond our limitations.

13.21. May God bless you for this good work. May your pupils now enjoy the beauty of yoga, and let them work hard to drink the nectar of yoga.

13.22. The eyes are closed, head is kept straight, eyes are drawn down and then back to seek "the One who is the True Light illuminating everyone." The hands are joined in front of the chest to greet the Lord who is inside. The mind is led to surrender to the very Soul within.

13.23. When the concrete is silent, then only can you go to the abstract. But many people want to go to the abstract without knowing the concrete.

13.24. *To D, who asked him about clearing up all the little troubles he was feeling:* My dear friend, don't take marks of weakness as if they were marks of spiritual advancement. Eat better, work better, and your marks of spiritual advancement will disappear.

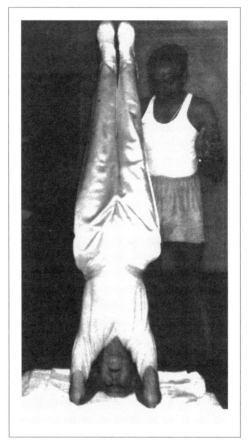

IYENGAR WITH QUEEN ELIZABETH OF BELGUIM IN SIRSASANA

13.25. Whatever you may do, do it completely, with body, mind, spirit, and in complete beauty and purity.

13.26. The important thing is to do what we are doing and not to think of what we have to do.

13.27. Don't teach only to teach. Teach to improve the student. To be a teacher requires vigorous discipline of one's own self.

13.28. The work of the pupil is to adjust his body to the words of the teacher.

13.29. You must savor the fragrance of a posture. Until you are relaxed, you cannot savor the fragrance.

13.30. Rhythm has to be observed in yoga more than staying.

13.31. As long as the body is not held firm, meditation is impossible, because the movement of the body is a disturbance of the intellect.

13.32. Intelligence has to be trained for the dull part of the body and not for the intelligent part.

13.33. The brain should be supple; the body should be as firm as a root.

13.34. The body should be held firm as a rock, and the brain should be as gentle, as subtle, as the thin ends of the leaves that move even in a gentle breeze.

13.35. Pain is unbearable; a stretch is bearable. We must know if we experience a bad pain or one that gives us a nice feeling.

13.36. You must keep the balance by the intelligence of the body (instinct, balance feeling, or ability) and not by strength. When you keep the balance by strength, it is physical action; when by intelligence of the body, it is relaxation in action.

13.37. Yoga is harmony of the body, senses, mind, and intellect. That's why there is no difference between physical and spiritual yoga.

13.38. When the chest opens, the mind opens, and we feel emotionally radiant, and stability comes. This is emotional stability.

13.39. *Upon Loustic's death (the small dog N's mother loved so much):* I am sorry to learn that you and your mother have lost your little dog. When such things happen, we must face them without losing heart. I hope that your mother is not too upset after the death of Loustic.

In Geneva he had said Loustic was a saint and would be reborn in a good man's body. One day, while eating, as Loustic was staring straight into his eyes, I asked Iyengar, "Is that ekagrata *(one-pointedness)?" His answer was:* "Yes, we have to look at the Lord with such intensity."

13.40. *During a pranayama class:* The sound is your guru.

13.41. When you do the posture with violence, I see violence in your face and in your practice.

13.42. What has a yogi to do with wealth? The wealth is within us. Our bodies and our minds are our wealth. First, let us utilize these.

1972

14.1. Nature has provided us with excellent capital—the body—to build up vast resources. The moment this body is neglected, education suffers.

14.2. Analysis in action—that is what yoga teaches you. Action of the body and analysis of the mind must be synchronized. This synchronization brings harmonious development.

14.3. Firmness in the body leads to firmness in the nervous system.

14.4. A perfect body is the only fit instrument for God to dwell in.

14.5. When the consciousness of the brain (the intellectual body) is brought to the consciousness of the mind (the mental or emotional body) they are encased (enclosed) in one another—then the Soul shines.

14.6. When the brain and the mind are silent, one experiences the consciousness of the self.

14.7. Yoga is Self-realization through the understanding of the body.

14.8. Think of God and remember Him.

14.9. The first five steps of yoga, if nurtured with care, will prepare the body, the mind, and the intellect to serve as fit vehicles for spiritual growth. And it has to end in the final absorption into the Infinite, which is its true purpose and natural end.

14.10. God is regarded as half man and half woman (*Ardhanarisvara*), representing the masculine and feminine manifestation in nature. Man and woman are regarded as God, and marriage is considered as a holy union of man and woman to form a divine Whole.

14.11. F still has three years to become a woman; she has to choose. The mind should not be allowed to wander. It is the age of determination—not struggle, only determination.

14.12. In the process of yoga, due to heightened circulation and breathing, you can explore the very remote ends of the nerves, so that they become completely healthy and sensitive and without tension. And when there is no tension in action, knowledge comes by itself, love by itself. Many of us work, but not with the right spirit, the spirit of love, of going completely into something, totally.

The practice of yoga makes you go deep into your actions, which saves your energy because your work-time is reduced due to the purification of your circulatory and respiratory systems. This is why we can face the challenge of keeping peace in the modern world.

14.13. Yoga has some techniques by which the senses are drawn to their source and thereby made free from desire. This gives mental stability, which is very essential for intellectual clarity, alertness, sharpness, and agility. Such an alert and agile mind can dispose of the day's work with ease and quick dispatch. It also eliminates tension.

14.14. All may be fit to do yoga, but only one in a million is fit to be called a yogi.

14.15. It is good to show what refinement means. Patanjali says that there are seven types of awareness. It is hard to explain, but as a layman, I say: physical awareness, physiological awareness, mental awareness, ethical awareness (which brings purity), intellectual awareness, awareness of refinement (in one's actions and behavior), awareness of the very Soul. These are the ways to observe while doing yoga.

14.16. Yoga is life-abundant and not life-negation. It is the only system I know of which develops harmoniously both the brawn and the brain.

14.17. Yesterday I told my pupils, "The maximum of what you did yesterday becomes the minimum of today."

14.18. The culture of the body is culture of the Self. The body is the temple of the Spirit. A yogi has to go further; for a yogi, the body is a fit temple for the Lord to dwell in only when it is completely virtuous (Upanishads). The Lord will enter the body only when total discipline, intellectual and ethical, is there.

14.19. Don't discuss with your pupils; don't waste your time.

14.20. Yoga is an art which disciplines and develops the body, the emotions, and the intellectual faculties, its purpose being to refine man.

14.21. When you know your body perfectly, the infinite is yours, because your mind is free from the entanglements of the body.

14.22. The extremities of the body should be nearer the Soul. The Soul exists everywhere; it is not localized, as the intelligence is localized in the brain. From the sockets, penetrate the intellect, following the sound through the ears, not the sound of the breath but the sound of the vibration of the consciousness within, the sound of your own existence, there where it originates, so that the brain is completely encased within the very existence of your Self. This is not a relaxation, but a discipline of evenness within.

14.23. Health is not a facility; it is a perfect balance between the body, the mind, and the soul. To obtain health, we need to know the nerves.

14.24. Yoga is a subject that has to be experienced, not merely discussed or argued about. Even if one wants to discuss it or argue about it, one has to experience it, because what one experiences is direct knowledge, and it is the imprint left from this direct knowledge that makes discussion possible. If the experience does not coordinate with the mental image or thinking about the experience, then either the experience is insufficient or the thinking over of the experience is not precise. When both tally, that is factual or direct knowledge. That is yoga.

14.25. Education, derived from the Latin *educare*, means to educe or draw forth or unfold the latent or potential—that is, to develop the talents and gifts of the individual. In short, it is the drawing out of the best qualities of a person. It is the task of a good educator to help his students realize their strength or their weakness, and then contribute to their growth and development on the one hand and eradication of weakness on the other. Unfortunately, nowadays instruction given in schools and colleges to enable a student to pass an examination is often confused with the term *education* and is also mistaken as a license to obtain employment and to earn one's livelihood.

14.26. We all speak of health. It is not a commodity that you swallow in the form of drugs and pills. It is a perfect state of equilibrium between the body, the mind, and soul, and that equilibrium destroys the duality within us. The effect of yoga is felt when the purity of knowledge is kindled in you. To gain health, you have to know the unconscious mind, which expresses itself within our nervous system. If the nerves are disturbed, then you feel the weakness of your mind. As long as the nerves are strong, stable, and elastic, so also the mind is stable.

14.27. Do not let the present stagnate; let it move towards purity.

14.28. Unless you know A, you can't learn B. So also in yoga, there are steps. Hatha Yoga is not physical yoga but a yoga of will and self power. It is a positive, straight, and difficult path; it is knowledge of the will, not physical yoga.

14.29. *In front of one of the neolithic polished stones of the Museum of National Antiquities in St. Germain-en-Laye:* "How many years, and how many men were needed to make this stone so smooth?" He passed his finger over one of the furrows, and after that, touched the huge stone to feel the difference, and went on, "How many years are required for a man to become as polished as this furrow?" E asked, "Is one life sufficient?" He answered that it was not sufficient, and for that there is reincarnation.

14.30. The body, like a boat, carries the indweller, the soul, from the shores of bondage to the shores of liberation. Liberation is, after all, freedom from the entanglements of both body and senses.

14.31. Pain and suffering force us to take cognizance of our body.

14.32. Yoga leads to a state in which life and death are one.

14.33. Attracted to a life of pleasure, the individual begins to believe that such pleasures are eternal, whereas in fact they are merely transitory. Caught in the giddy whirl of pleasures, he is blinded and fails to see this. A discriminating person, however, sees through the ephemeral veil of sensory pleasures and learns to channel the outgoing energy of the senses inward. He turns that energy back to the shrine of the Divinity, the Soul.

14.34. If something goes wrong with the body, the temple of the Soul, then the ultimate goal, which is God-realization through Self-realization, cannot be reached.

14.35. The Kathopanishad by an apt comparison reminds us that the body is important in the spiritual quest. It compares the body to a chariot, the senses to horses, the mind to the reins. The intellect is the charioteer, and the *jivatma* (individual soul) is the master of the chariot. But let something go wrong with the chariot, or the horses, or the reins, or the charioteer, and not only the chariot and charioteer but also the master will come to grief.

14.36. The aphorisms of Patanjali make it easy for us to estimate the value of yoga as a fount of Self-realization, enclosing within itself the three paths of *karma*, *jnana*, and *bhakti*. The three are closely intermingled and interrelated.

14.37. The body, the temple of the Soul, should be neither neglected nor pampered. For it is the only instrument and the only resource we are provided with to meet our Creator, the Lord. It may be fashionable to despise the body as something nonspiritual, yet none can afford to neglect it. The moment we neglect or pamper it, attachment to it increases, and the right royal road to *Atma-darsan* (Self-realization) is lost.

14.38. For the improvement of the self, four paths were laid down by the great sages of the world: path of knowledge, path of love, path of action, path of yoga. Intelligence is a part of knowledge. Emotion is a part of love. The body with its vehicles, its arms, legs, members, is a part of action. And to acquire pure action, to experience pure love, and to have that quality of wisdom, the path of yoga is the fountain.

14.39. As T feels completely lost, she gets a lot of courage and surrenders completely. As you don't suffer, you protect yourselves, and you don't surrender.

14.40. The standing poses are meant to strengthen the ankles and the knees. When people are mentally disturbed, dejected, you'll notice they can't stand firmly on their feet. These postures teach one how to stand straight, so that the brain can stay in its place. It is like the roots of the tree. If you can't stand properly on your feet, you develop a negative approach. These postures help you to maintain stability in times of catastrophe.

14.41. The two last steps of the Yoga Sutras are states of oneness, wherein body-mind and mind-soul dualities vanish, and the seeker becomes an integrated personality who has no feeling of I or me or mine. That is yoga.

14.42. Father X suggested that I should make a pilgrimage to the Vatican to have an audience with His Holiness Pope Paul VI. This suggestion left me dumb. His Holiness is considered by the Christian world as the direct descendant of St. Peter, who was a close friend and disciple of Jesus. How on earth is it possible for a non-Christian mortal like me to have this most enviable audience, I wondered. God blessed the God on earth to grant me the audience, and the gates of God of heaven would open to me, as the doors of the God on earth opened.

We reached Castel Gandolfo, the summer residence of the head of the Christian world. Thousands and thousands thronged the Castel to get a glimpse of the Holy Father. The gatherings there are like many sacred places in India, where thousands and thousands gather for *darsan* in temples on important occasions.

We went near the Castel gates, and two guards stopped us at the gate and asked for the appointment letter. I presented the letter, and they allowed me to enter. I asked for my friend's admission. They flatly refused, as the audience was for me only. So I had to leave my friend behind, though my heart was sore.

I found a big assembly hall, or *darbar*. People from various parts of the globe came to have the darsan of the Holy Father. In a few seconds, my eyes glittered to gaze at a man—the great Pope—with long yellow robes and a white cap on his head. Thus ended my momentous journey to the holy city of Rome, where God's chosen representative lives.

14.43. When the brain is active, the mind wakes up as an intelligence, in the seat of the brain. When the brain is perfectly quiet and the center of the intellect is in peace, then we are at the same time together with ourselves and floating, empty, and yet perfectly satisfied. Serene, balanced, neither free nor bound, we find quietness in a pure consciousness, because the intelligence is in its source, the mind.

14.44. Faith, courage, and intelligent and uninterrupted awareness—these qualities are to be present whether one is wide awake, half asleep, or in deep slumber. An individual who lives like this performs his daily actions with a mind free from selfishness. This is poise in action. And this poise leads to that serenity which is in the truest sense a healthy mind in a healthy body.

14.45. I do my best and am contented with it.

14.46. The instrument of the self is the body. Unless the intelligence of the body is transmitted to the intellect or the mind, quietness within is impossible. The state of Self-realization is an experience of oneness within one's own self in the discipline of yoga. There are several impediments that come in the way of this realization. And we have to work very hard to keep these impediments from getting in our way, so that the intelligence is free from the attachment of the body and the emotions, so that it can be one with the Spirit or the Soul within.

14.47. One gradually masters the art of keeping the mind in a zero position, i.e., observing that the energy of the body is not dissipated but adjusted and retained within the body.

14.48. Yoga is harmony of the body, of the senses, of the spirit, and of the intellect. This is why there is no difference between physical yoga and spiritual yoga.

14.49. The pose is not a rigid state in quietness which, although it cuts you off from the outside world, remains egoistic. Savasana, when it is correctly done, brings interior peace and calm silence, which is divine.

14.50. Spiritual knowledge begins when the mind extends a little further than where it is at present.

14.51. In Savasana, the ego consciousness is merged with the creator consciousness. Emotional stability and mental humility are there.

14.52. We have to face; we should face.

14.53. Precision in action is yoga. The Lord is Precision.

14.54. As intelligence develops in you, so you must also try and have a synchronization of mind and body. As long as they are not synchronized, there is a duality: the duality of mind and body, mind and intellect, intellect and soul.

14.55. Awareness is attention that is watching, whether attention is here, there, or everywhere.

14.56. In pranayama, the head is bent onto the chest with a chin-lock that quiets the heart and leads to the peaceful center where the Lord dwells.

14.57. By inspiration we receive our life from God. Retention is sweet to the Lord, in the peaceful depth of the heart. Exhalation is the highest form of surrendering to the Lord.

14.58. The brain must be flexible, the body must be as rigid as stone. When the brain is perfectly calm, then meditation begins.

14.59. Yoga gives complete stability and integrates body, mind, intellect, and consciousness. This, in short, is *Atma-darsan*, or Self-enlightenment.

14.60. Take each pore of the skin for a conscious eye. Adjust and balance gently your body from inside with the help of these conscious eyes, as it is difficult for normal eyes (the external ones) to observe and correct the body position (adjusting it from both sides).

14.61. When in meditation, look with your ears, not with your eyes. When you look with your eyes, the brain is aggressive (that is, when you concentrate on an object with the energy concentrated in the frontal brain, where the eyes are). When you look with the ears, the brain in silent. Ears bring the art of silence. Eyes bring the art of action. When one understands this, one knows the art of meditation.

14.62. We have forgotten the very education of the body, and yet we want something more, beyond!

14.63. Yoga leads to the transparence of wisdom through the education of the spirit, of the will, of the soul, and of the body.

14.64. For me, yoga is character building—the development of a character that ensures unity and harmony of the body, the mind, and the soul—a well-integrated, mature personality at peace with itself and with society.

14.65. Yoga embraces everything. To consider it as purely physical is as wrong as calling it purely spiritual. It embraces the physical aspect, the physiological aspect, the psychological aspect, and the spiritual aspect, too. It starts with the cultivation of the body, as we have to use that alone as a guiding star to improve our consciousness. So yoga is all; it is to develop the wisdom of the body as well as the wisdom of the intellect. This is my way of yoga—an integrated science that has taught me to live from the body to the soul and from the soul to the body.

14.66. The posture should be comfortable and steady, says Patanjali. But that steadiness comes only when the effort has ended. So you have to train the body, so that the complex becomes simple. There is no strain anywhere; my effort has ceased. Because my effort has ceased, one is one with the Infinite.

14.67. Yoga is not an intellectual game; it's a part of real experience.

14.68. It is not mere quietness but the renunciation of our ego and conscious receptivity to the divinity we carry within ourselves.

14.69. As long as my children are not married, I conform strictly to the rules of my community.

14.70. It is less difficult to acquire something than to keep it, because we become proud and do not practice any longer, so we lose what we acquired and lose humility, as well.

14.71. When my mind, my body, my senses enjoy a certain action and my mind says it is enough, it is at that point that spiritual *sadhana* begins. This is spiritual tranquility. So also in breathing, you have to learn the ethical discipline of physical respiration, and if that principle is lost, the intellectual and ethical discipline is gone and we do it mechanically, and that mechanical practice is not spiritual sadhana. When something becomes mechanical, it is no longer a spiritual sadhana. You must recharge your batteries. It is similar to the flow of uninterrupted intelligence. That is yoga.

14.72. When walking, extend the body towards the brain without shaking the brain.

14.73. An ethical diet is to eat as long as saliva comes in your mouth when seeing a meal, and to stop at the very moment it doesn't come.

14.74. In pranayama, when you inhale, do not disturb the position of the consciousness of the brain or the eyes or the eyelids. Let them explore or see into the lungs and into the spine. Then you will understand what I said.

14.75. *At the Museum of Saint Germain-en-Laye, in front of a big, round urn, I say, "Kumbhaka (retention)."*
    "Yes," he says, "*Kumbha*. When it is completely full, there is no more vibration, no more noise."

14.76. Real *kumbhaka* is at the top of the chest, not here *(he touches his floating ribs)*, always at the top. It should push by the inner edge of the ribs, not by the exterior edge. Kumbhaka should be done by the inner edge. How can I explain more unless I see your pupil? If I see him, I can tell you.

14.77. The ribs are the wings of the body. Open your wings.

14.78. I have also been branded in England as rough, violent, proud, and so on, a yogi without yogic manners, but they claim as well that I am the only best teacher. How can all that go together?

Precision and perfection are ruthless. In that ruthless teaching and practice, the fineness shines. Very few understand the severity of yoga. A straight path is a hard path. But all want comfort.

14.79. If the breathing is defective, the intelligence cannot function, because there is no way energy can be taken in.

14.80. As long as I serve my pupils, I consider my pupils as my God.

14.81. Determined effort alone leads to the goal.

14.82. In asana, the eyes should be active. When you do the breathing, the ears should be active. The eyes cannot penetrate the mind because it is a vibration. The mind is in space; the brain is not in space. The mind is a gross form of consciousness. So whenever you feel the intelligence, the mind is active. The brain thinks, but it does not penetrate. The sound of the mind is a vibration that can be perceived only by the ears.

14.83. Children have to learn how to face things. You must not cry when seen. Out of ten persons seeing you crying, there will be ten various explanations, and this will bring confusion. What is the use of this weeping? It does not solve the problem. It increases sorrow. Every time sorrow comes, you must close the problem, end the chapter; then strength comes. Sorrow allows you to be receptive to the Divinity.

14.84. *In answer to a question about how to place the mat, which direction to face, to do yoga:* I sanctify the place where I work by yoga.

14.85. Asceticism is not to hold at any cost a pose that is painful, but to do this very pose with as much intensity of intelligence and love as possible.

14.86. You should never allow the mind to wander. If you expect to gather super sensitivities, you destroy yourself. God blesses those who walk following a straight line. A straight line is a difficult one, but it brings its own fruits; it's the only constructive one.

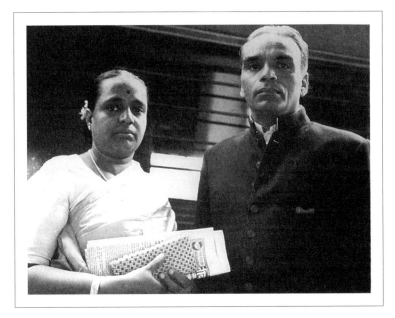

RAMAMANI AND B.K.S. IYENGAR, 1963

1973

15.1. Though we are affected by the loss of my wife, I have to take it calmly, as I have so much responsibility to bear.

15.2. *Is yoga exclusively Indian?*

Can any science accept such narrow thinking? Is there American electricity or Russian cancer or European tuberculosis? Yoga is for all men, women, and children, irrespective of race, color, sex, language, or religion. Yoga, after all, aims at a union of individual consciousness with cosmic or universal consciousness. In this sense, yoga as a way of thinking, feeling, and living is truly international. To limit yoga to the boundaries of one nation in these days of moon landing is the denial of universal cosmic consciousness.

15.3. What X said about me is both truth and untruth. So the world moves, equally balancing truth and untruth. May God bless him. I am not hurt at all, but I see what a human mind is made up of. Convey my greetings to him.

15.4. Like anatomy, yoga is a practical science dealing with human development. There is no question of miracles. What appears as a miracle to an ordinary person might be the manifestation of an established law in the realm of nature. Miracles have their own value in rousing the curiosity of men. However, sage Patanjali, the father of yoga, warns the student of yoga of the dangers of *siddhi*, or the power to work miracles.

Walking on water, swallowing nails, and such other feats are all possible. These powers are the result of certain specific *sadhana*. But these are all passing phases in the process of man's development as an integrated being. It is the maturity of body, nerves, emotions, and intellect which is important in acquiring perfect Consciousness.

15.5. *Please teach us the technique of Transcendental Meditation.*

Meditation is one. There is, according to me, no such thing as Transcendental Meditation. Raising of consciousness from one set of conditionings to another is the object of meditation. When all conditioning ceases to operate for the meditator (the subject), then there is no meditator separate from the object (of meditation). The postures for meditation are simple, either Padmasana or Sukhasana, where the eyes are drawn towards the seat of the mind (the heart center), with the spine erect and the brain quiet. This transformation from one to the other is called transcendental because you are transcending from one state to the other. (*Transcend* comes from an Indo-European root *skand* = he jumps.)

15.6. *Is celibacy essential for practicing yoga?*

I myself am a married man and father of six children; that should answer your question.

15.7. *What about dietary discipline?*

Geography has much to do with diet. Climate and other such factors influence the diet of people. But here are some basic guidelines. Do not eat if saliva does not spring from the mouth when food is brought before you. Secondly, when the brain alone speculates about the choice of food, it means the body does not need food. Even then, if you eat, it will not be nourishing. It will be an abuse of food.

15.8. *Have you Beatles and hippies as your followers?*
No. When they see the discipline that I demand in my class, they go away.

15.9. *After his wife's death:* God has to give me strength to put up with the strain after the loss of my dearest. I have now no one with whom to share my feelings, and yoga is my only solace.

15.10. All these years I was a *sannyasi* with a wife. Now I am a householder without a wife.

15.11. *From an obituary of Ramamani, Iyengar's wife:* Her main aim in life was to serve and protect her husband in his yoga *sadhana* and in his teaching. For her, the husband was God. She drank the nectar of Divinity through him.

15.12. *Are you a hatha yogi or a raja yogi?*
I am neither a hatha yogi nor a raja yogi. I am only a yoga practitioner. It is not correct to demarcate yoga into such artificial divisions as *karma, bhakti,* and *jnana* except for theoretical purposes. The word *hatha* is composed of two letters, *ha* and *tha. Ha* is the sun, or positive electricity, and *tha* is negative electricity, or the moon. The union of the two generates bioenergy. That science is hatha yoga.

Raja means "king" or "soul." Raja yoga also leads to Self-realization. Yoga as such is the science of an integrated, balanced personality in which the intellect and the emotions are well blended.

15.13. I think the will to do is the summum bonum of yoga. As one progresses in yoga, character also improves. Fundamentally, what is required is tenacity of purpose, determination to work hard, and complete faith in what one does.

15.14. *Is yoga a science or art?*

Yoga is both. Where there is a technique, there is science. Yoga has its own technique of physiological, psychological, and supramental well-being of man. Like a musician who plays his instrument, the student or adept in yoga plays with his body, depicting various animate forms of nature. Like a sculptor fashioning out a sculpture, the yogi chisels his body and mind and expands his consciousness into the universe.

If you accept the view that there is no art without philosophy, yoga is also a kind of philosophy, in which the practitioner is drawn to the shrine of divinity within himself. It is the art of living truly. Yoga does not express a view on life. Rather it is a way towards right living. Hence it is a science, an art, and a philosophy. Yoga is a science of character building or right conduct.

1974

16.1. You can use the word *Soul* for the larger Self or Overself. Ego is the small self. "I" or "me," the pronoun, is the small self. To go beyond is Soul.

16.2. Without morality there is no religion, and without religion no morality. They are like the two wings of a bird that can fly; with one wing, it cannot fly. So both are essential. The end of religion is Self-knowledge, Self-realization. Morality is the shore of one side of the river to take you to the other shore of the river, called *dharma*. *Dharma* has no English equivalent; that which upholds, sustains, and supports the Soul is religion.

16.3. *What about your apparent anger in the classes?*

As long as my anger is not destructive, it is building you up. I want to break the inertia in you. If anger continues in your system when it is over, the anger is destructive. When anger dissolves in itself, it is not destructive. Destructive anger is one that penetrates the self continuously. Patanjali said, You must be as hard as a diamond, as soft as a rose petal.

Look at the word *ahimsa*, which rules on how to behave in society. Have I done any harm to you? The doctor who removes your sick organs, why don't you tell him not to be violent? Patanjali said, Intensity alone will bring a man more quickly to the end. He has given three different qualities of students: mild, moderate, intense.

The important question in regard to my apparent anger is how to break the lethargy in the beginning. It's just like working with someone who takes drugs. First of all you must help them find their psychological balance, and then the drugs will drop off automatically.

16.4. Extension brings freedom.

16.5. The whole body has to act. To extend a part, you must extend the whole.

16.6. When the mind is stable, then the physical comes.

16.7. Everything should be symmetrical; that is why yoga is a basic art.

16.8. *Hatha* means "will," so you must use your will. Using your will with intelligence in everything you do. It means stubbornness.

16.9. As the potter uses his hands to mold the pot, so should you use your zeal to mold yourself.

16.10. In the struggle alone, there is knowledge.

16.11. How to project the intelligence from the source? The intelligence shouldn't be broken. Can the intelligence be kept in the head and projected into the back, and then into the lumbar region?

16.12. Awareness is subjective attention without frontier, without boundary, without limitation. Concentration is to get focused on a point, on an object.

16.13. There should always be a certain amount of pain; then only will you see the light.

16.14. The intelligence extends with the movement of the body. That is maturity.

16.15. As long as you cannot move your skin, you are all egoists.

16.16. As long as you are living in the Self, you are coming close to immortality.

16.17. To get freedom from fear, you must face pain. Freedom comes only when you are desireless. The end of discipline is the beginning of freedom. Discipline must become second nature. You must do it but not worry about it. You must reach that state of divine vision (*mukta*), where to live in the Self is freedom.

16.18. You must purge yourself before finding fault in others.

16.19. *Atma-darsan* is experience of the Self. It is the same as Patanjali's third *sloka* of the first chapter: "Then the seer comes to consciousness of his proper nature."

16.20. One who lives totally in the body lives totally in the Self.

16.21. Pain prevents the self from flowing further, as our attention is interrupted. We must convert unbearable pain to bearable pain, so we must touch the nerves before touching the mind.

16.22. God has blessed me beyond my capacity in yoga. How far I have advanced, I do not know. I only know that I am doing better and that I am clear in my practices.

16.23. *Is old age postponed by the control of the breath?*
Death is certain. Why worry about it? Let it come when it comes. Just keep working. The Self has no age. It doesn't die. Only the body decays. The moment you don't take care of your garden, it dries up.

16.24. In the Upanishads it is said: You have to train the body for the spirit to enter.

16.25. The exterior and the interior meet in an inner balance.

16.26. The inner gaze must be in the center. If consciousness is in either one of the feet, the posture goes off balance.

16.27. Balance equals spiritual attainment.

16.28. *Sadhana* is *abhyasa* (practice). A *sadhaka* is one who does abhyasa. Abhyasa covers all the aspects of yoga in general and in particular the first *sloka* of the second chapter of Patanjali: "Their aim is to bring soul-vision and to wear away hindrances."

16.29. God bless those who are honest in the subject they love.

16.30. The river when it joins the sea does not say, "I'm joining the sea"; it is obvious. So the mind does not say, "I am joining the Self."

16.31. *Samadhi* is where everything is stilled, where you are completely conscious.

16.32. As the river runs evenly when full, so our intelligence must go like a full river.

16.33. There are two kinds of knowledge: *vidya*, acquired knowledge, and *buddhi*, knowledge which comes from your own action and experience in life. There is also *pramana*, which is indirect perception, and experience, which is direct perception.

16.34. In meditation, there is no object to look upon, to depend on. Instead, you become one with the object, so that the object is transformed into the subject. Like the river that does not claim to be running, flowing, but it is one from the mountain to the sea. Meditation is like that. If you measure the distance from mountain to sea, and concentrate on that distance, it has a point, space, area; that is concentration, not meditation.

16.35. The posture should describe the quality of *prashanta* (peace and poise), the flow of energy like the river. Movement without interruption.

16.36. *What about pain when doing yoga?*
      When you begin yoga, the unrecognized pains come to the surface. When

the *prakriti* has ascended to the level of the soul, then the hidden pains are dispersed.

16.37. *Can a paralyzed person do yoga?*
   A paralyzed person accepts his disease; his mind doesn't put tension in his body. He is free to think about God.

16.38. Yoga makes an extrovert from an introvert, and an introvert from an extrovert.

16.39. *Can you do yoga and still be an atheist?*
   If you believe in perfection, you believe in Divinity. Yoga has a scientific background. If you use the word *perfection* in speaking of yoga, then anybody can do it.

16.40. "Put your brain in your knee" means pay attention, or bring your intelligence to act in that place.

16.41. It's better to learn ten poses very well, that way you enjoy the fruit of your work. I never go ahead as long as there is confusion in one of the poses.

16.42. Pain is your guru.

16.43. We must translate physical action into spiritual action.

16.44. The body has to say, "I can do it," not the intellect. There should be a complete understanding between the mind and the body.

16.45. *How does yoga affect religion?*

Yoga is greater than the culture of the self, which is involved in having an ethical standard based on certain religious doctrines.

16.46. The body is relaxed when the brain is relaxed.

16.47. You live to die, to give your life for others. This requires five qualities: courage, vitality, memory, awareness, and becoming absorbed in what another is trying to do.

16.48. *On the divine marriage between nature and consciousness:* When consciousness comes in contact with nature, nature changes.

16.49. Learning is as much an art as teaching.

16.50. The brain receives and acts at the same time.

16.51. For you, yoga is outside of you. For me, it's inside. For you, it's only a thing.

16.52. Every yogi says we should not strain, but do you know how much you strain in other areas?

16.53. The intelligence should be everywhere. Your intelligence is only in the brain; that is why you're suffering.

16.54. You must bring the unconscious into the conscious. Intensified action brings intensified intelligence, says Patanjali.

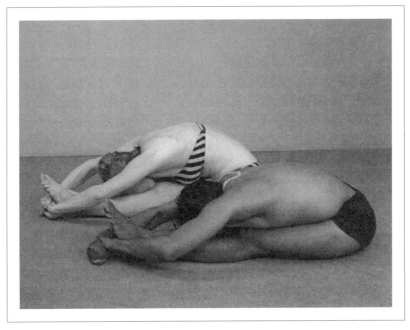

IYENGAR AND NOËLLE IN PASCHIMOTTANASANA

16.55. If you know the fountain, then knowledge is there forever.

16.56. It requires tremendous concentration to let the energy flow from the feet. Then you are near the Self.

16.57. Yoga is a physiological exercise that should be converted into psychological action.

16.58. Pupils should be self-aware, not self-conscious.

16.59. When one is in a meditative state, the frontal brain is resting, and the back of the brain is acting. The awareness should flow without interruption. If there is interruption, you must charge the battery. Then the unconscious and conscious are one.

16.60. You have to create love and affection for your body.

16.61. You should know how to relax in action.

16.62. When something new and better comes without learning it, it is as quick as the dried leaves falling from the tree.

16.63. The brain is the receiving instrument. We must make the adjustment in the brain in a split second.

16.64. Self-protection is not selfishness. It is also a form of spiritual knowledge.

16.65. All parts of the body should be aware. All should be in relation to the Self. Everything should be in contact. You must look for nonduality in the posture. This can be done by keeping everything in touch with the Self. All movement begins from the Self.

16.66. If the foundation is firm, the building can withstand anything. Yoga is the foundation that allows the self to be converted into the subject.

16.67. The mind always plays a dual role between the body and the self. It wants to please the senses and the self. The mind is a bottomless pit; it is always full of desires. But if you get to the bottom, there is no more desire.

16.68. The body is the only concrete instrument on which you can concentrate. It frees the rest to become introverted and meditative.

16.69. If you have observed something, you can also feel it.

16.70. One man has done it, so you can do it.

16.71. Freedom is to be free from fear, to be desireless.

16.72. When you have learned to stretch completely, you have learned to relax completely.

16.73. We have two physical eyes, but every pore of the body is also an eye.

16.74. The receiving intellect is the meditative intellect.

16.75. Yoga is meditation: having reached the highest fragrance in one's intellectual standard, and retaining that peak of intelligence and understanding, to keep the mind in a state of perpetual innocence.

16.76. *Does one have to be a celibate to do yoga?*
Yoga is practiced to keep one free from desires and still live fully. In the olden days, everyone was a householder, but they followed a certain principle: sex was a spiritual act. The license to act as you like is not freedom. A celibate is he who does not indulge in sex too often.

16.77. We begin with the physical, then we forget it. One must discipline the mind through action.

16.78. *What happens when you feel pain in doing a posture?*

There are two kinds of pain: physical and mental. If you have a pain that persists and intensifies as you work, it's an indication that it's wrong. But you must be pliable intellectually. The advanced classes give pain. You must face it.

16.79. The known is limited, but the unknown is vast. Go more and more to the unknown. The moment you touch it, it becomes known and also limited.

16.80. The mind is not balanced when you force.

16.81. The breath is superior to the mind. If you understand how to distribute the *prana,* you can make the energies of the individual and the universal meet.

16.82. *At what point should one do pranayama?*

Patanjali has not given any steps except the relationship between asana and pranayama, which should be practiced when you have perfected the postures. If your attention is not perfectly mastered in the cells of your body, how can you let the breath penetrate everywhere?

16.83. In this world, words without action are considered enough.

16.84. We must free the mind from the attachment of the body. The body is the kingdom of the self. The self should move freely in our body to the extreme pores of the skin.

16.85. Do from your mind, not from your brain. Spiritual knowledge comes from the mind.

16.86. Rhythm has to be observed in yoga.

16.87. Whatever one is doing, one should do it as an offering to God.

16.88. The regimented training of yoga keeps the mind alert.

16.89. *To pupils lined up waiting their turn to be taken in backbends:* I can see by the way you stand those who want to do and those who do not.

16.90. Awareness must flow uninterruptedly through the conscious state.

16.91. A posture can be considered as much as a mantra or as much as meditation.

16.92. Yoga is the music of the body, the mind, and the soul, because these three are all in unison.

16.93. The body is the temple of the spirit. Let the temple be clean through yoga.

16.94. When pain is persistent or increased, then the action is wrong. Self-protection is also spiritual knowledge.

16.95. The aftereffects of sedatives and all drugs create an unbalanced mind.

16.96. Yoga is the music of the soul. So continue, and the gates of the soul will open.

16.97. To achieve the end of yoga, uninterrupted practice is demanded.

16.98. The balance of the mind is rocked if one uses force.

16.99. Selfishness means rigidity. Selflessness means pliability.

16.100. The instrument, the body, must be pure. The instrument of recognition, the mind, must be trained to be in contact with the Self.

16.101. Your bodies are in the past; your minds in the future. When you do yoga, they come together in the present.

16.102. Trust in yoga as I do, and practice regularly.

16.103. Love, labor, and laugh.

16.104. When the object, the instrument of recognition of the object, and the recognizer are one, then that is meditation.

16.105. Your body is the child of the soul. You must nourish and train your child.

16.106. Freedom is precision, and yoga takes me there.

16.107. Your brains are stung by the poison of the scorpion; the scorpion is vanity.

16.108. The philosophy of pain is to conquer.

16.109. Intelligence must be like the rays of the sun—extending everywhere, penetrating all.

16.110. You people are so dull! You cannot work and you cannot relax.

16.111. The single eye is the Self. The single mind is a pure mind; it has no beginning, it has no end.

16.112. When you exceed your limitations, then the gates of the mind open.

16.113. Activity is not tension. Tension is oscillation. Meditation is the imitation of deep sleep in the wakeful state.

16.114. You are too intelligent. Can you not be intelligently intelligent?

16.115. I love you, that is why I hate you when you don't work.

16.116. Think of God in all that you do whether it is yoga or outside yoga. That is a step of *Atma sadhana.* God is concrete and absolute. You can think of Him in a form or in a new idea or in new creations. They are all part of Him.

16.117. *To a class who had incurred his displeasure:* You people are so easy to deceive. I'll come back next year as the guru Maharaj, all sweetness and love, and you will think, what a wonderful teacher. And afterwards, what will you have when I have gone?

16.118. Position God in Paschimottanasana on the floor, in Sarvangasana on the ceiling, and in Sirsasana in front. That way you can think of the inflow and outflow of breath in *kumbhaka* as though His entire being has entered your entire body.

16.119. In Savasana, the jaws, the eyes, the muscles of the face, eyebrows, forehead, all have to sink backward. In the beginning, draw the eyes towards the emotional center and feel the grip. Then, retaining the organic grip, the muscles of the eyes should be relaxed. Do not open the mouth in order to relax; in the beginning only, to understand better, open the lips, release the jaws, and then close the lips without tightening the jaws.

16.120. Men and women have some weak points. When dedicated, devoted practice is maintained, these weaknesses dissolve as the intellectual plane reaches finer consciousness.

16.121. Hearsay is not knowledge.

16.122. Everything should be like a *sutra* knotted together in relationship to the center.

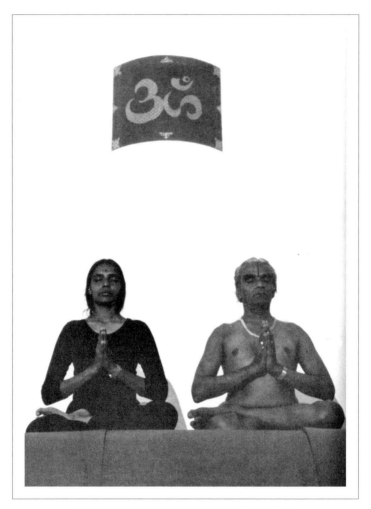

GEETA AND IYENGAR IN MEDITATION, PUNE, 1975

1975

17.1. Even the little toe has to work to retain its awareness.

17.2. Break bad habits and cultivate good habits to make progress.

17.3. Venture from the known into the unknown.

17.4. Why do you live in memory? Memory is useless if you repeat the past; memory is necessary if you use it to develop. If repetition is taking place, then that memory retards the path of evolution. Memory is only the vehicle to be used to know whether we are aware. Pursue, find out. Do not live in memory. Repetition means to live in memory. Memory is necessary to see whether we are receding or proceeding.

17.5. Go from the finite to the infinite; then you will experience no beginning, no end.

17.6. Keep the eyes open. Conquer the body before you close your eyes. When your eyes are open, you are aware. If you close your eyes without mastering yoga, you go into a blind state. Awareness must come with open eyes. You must learn to see behind you. When you are clear, perfection is obtained, then close the eyes and do. Then you are fully aware. Shutting your eyes means your mind is dull, you cannot see what is happening, cannot be aware. You use only your two physical eyes, that is why you are useless; use your intellectual eyes, too. To understand the world, you open your eyes. To understand the inside world, you close your eyes. This closing of the eyes should be followed only when one is stable both within and without.

17.7. A blind mind leads to a dreamy state.

17.8. When you place your mat on the floor, there is no duality. When you lower your head into position on the mat, there is no duality. But the moment you raise your feet from the floor, you experience the identity of "I." Take that away and retain the oneness, the total awareness which must remain throughout the posture.

17.9. Do not teach what you do not know. Before interpreting and experimenting on your students, learn and interpret on your own body.

17.10. Meditation means to live or be in a primitive state, without ignorance but with innocence.

17.11. Indian brain, horizontal; Western brain, vertical. Indians are caught up in subjective intelligence. Westerners are caught up in objective intelligence. To work a part, work the whole. Easterners work from the mind. Westerners work from the intellect.

17.12. *When asked to explain the previous saying, Iyengar answered as follows:*

The intelligence of man works in two directions, emotional on one side and intellectual on the other side. In order to get qualifications, degrees, and success in a vocation, intellectual knowledge is necessary. In order to understand man to man, his problems such as pleasures and pains, sex, family, happiness, contentment, and so on, emotional intelligence is needed. The brain works on the intellectual side and the mind on the emotional side. In the West, even emotional problems are worked out intellectually, that is, by acquired knowledge which is objective. They should be solved with subjective knowledge, an understanding that comes from one's own experience when one is in the emotional situation.

Science has made human intelligence go further and further, without being broad-based. When you come across a country man, he is warm, affectionate, and embracing, whereas the sophisticated city man thinks only of himself, his survival, his satisfaction, with no care for his fellow being. This is what I meant.

To work a part of the body, you have to work the whole. So also in order to work the whole, you have to work each and every part individually as well as collectively. I have explained this often in person, and it is no good asking me to answer in a letter that is not even worth the cost of a stamp.

17.13. If you do not surrender to your guru, at least at the time of learning surrender. If not, the ego is responsible for that pride.

17.14. Unless the disciple gives up his ego and follows the guru's instruction, he cannot make any physical, mental, or spiritual progress.

17.15. You are part of the Universe. You are without beginning and without end.

17.16. Marriage is the union of two souls to live amicably with each other.

17.17. The capital we are born with is the human body, which lies unutilized by the great majority of us. This realization alone is enough to understand what ethics requires. If care is not taken of the only capital that God has blessed us with to see the Divine, we are not only immoral, but irreligious, too. The moment we pay respect and mend the body, morality and religion begin.

17.18. Awaken the dormant intelligence even in the minutest fiber. This will help the neighboring fibers to revitalize, to realize their functions, to act, to experience what you have created.

17.19. Develop the intelligence, and see that the intelligence of the Self radiates its whole frontier—the body—as the sun radiates all around equally and evenly when not covered by clouds.

17.20. There is a popular misconception that yoga is only for those who have power of concentration. But all of us are not so endowed. A careful study of the literature on yoga indicates that yoga can be practiced by anyone, whether he has a *kshipta* (wandering mind), *mudha* (forgetful mind), *vikshipta* (oscillating mind), *ekagrata* (one-pointed mind), or *niruddha* (restrained mind).

17.21. The science of yoga is vast, and progress therein seems agonizingly and disappointingly slow. But yoga helped me to overcome physical, mental, and spiritual obstacles, so that today I am sipping the nectar of yoga.

17.22. I will not say that I have completely mastered this art and science even today. Perfection eludes us, but this should not reduce our efforts. The more I work, the more insignificant my efforts appear to be. I have to be content with this divine discontent that drives me on.

17.23. In Savasana or in meditation, the light of the eyes is drawn towards the lotus of the heart, so that the seat of the intelligence of the head is brought into contact with the seat of the intelligence of the heart, which is called the mind. Thus one passes from the individualistic state of consciousness to the universal state of consciousness. It is the merging of the intellect of the brain with the intellect of the soul.

17.24. *When Mr. Sauvage died, Mr. Iyengar wrote to Alice, his widow:*
May the Lord of yoga give you strength to bear this personal loss. God calls you back when your job is done in this world. May you be saved from sorrow by the Lord. We share the same sorrow with you at this juncture.

17.25. As in married life, sense pleasures are the key to a happy life. I said I have given all satisfaction to my wife, so we lived in joy and peace.

17.26. When we look at something with intensity, this intensity lasts only a few seconds, then we do nothing more than look in the mirror of the mind. We must keep the initial intensity for a longer time. The mind reflects both the self and what is seen.

17.27. If your head is kept so that the brain is balanced, you are in the present. That is meditation.

17.28. *Pointing at two pupils:* See the dullness of their faces. This is tranquility of the senses only. There is no meditation here because there is no improvement.

17.29. *About pranayama:* Not bliss, but purity, truth.

17.30. If the chest is the mother and the air the child, with inhalation the mother lets her child come to her, and with exhalation she lets him go without following him but still protecting him.

17.31. Watch the rectitude of the head. The front brain must go towards the back brain. The back brain is the mother; the other is the child. The mother welcomes the child. Union.

17.32. In *kumbhaka*, you should not hold the breath, but the breath should hold you.

17.33. Always keep the back alert, alive, not dull.

17.34. The back is like a frame; the front body, the painting that it throws into relief.

17.35. *Regarding the shoulder blades of a back that is not right:* They are like eggs, so you have to cut the eggs off.

17.36. The unconscious is the negative strength. The conscious is the positive strength.

17.37. *Regarding the work of pranayama:* The back is a blackboard; the air comes to write; the mind holds the chalk.

17.38. The seeker, the seeking, and the object have to become one.

17.39. The subject, the pupil, and the guru all should be one.

17.40. The crown of the head, the center of the forehead, the root of the nose, the tip of the nose, the middle lips, the middle of the chin, the middle of the sternum should all be in one line. The right and the left have to meet in the center. That means you are completely in contact. If there is loose-ness, there is no contact at all; the self and the body have lost contact, so you learn nothing.

17.41. Wisdom or understanding and skill are brought together to function within you. How to adjust each and every movement in this way is an art. To use the word *art* without reaching that state of perfection has no meaning.

17.42. When you close your eyes, do not just close your eyes. The right and the left ears have to move inwards for the eyes to close. Do you follow? The inner ears of the right and left should move towards the eyes to close the eyes.

17.43. Ears receptive, ears passive.

17.44. As the wind blows, so the leaves move. As the wind blows, so your mind moves.

17.45. The art of sitting is to let the front body and the back body both be nonaggressive. The word is simple; you know what *nonaggressive* is, but you do not do it. This is the physical body, which is the known body. Your intelligence can understand what this body is because it is very concrete. But there is a central portion of the body, and the front body and the back body both have to meet exactly in the center. So the body here is just the central portion; it is known as the unknown body.

17.46. When you sit, first stability, then physical firmness.

17.47. The seat of the brain is the lower self. The seat of the heart is the higher Self. In the exhalation, do not close the seat of the higher Self. So the lower self, which we call selfishness, has to reach the Self that has no color, no form, no shape, no odor.

17.48. Keeping your body erect without tensing the skin, face the inner body, the body which is in contact with your soul. The inner body has to raise your body up.

17.49. As you are inhaling, you must learn to merge the seat of the ego, which you call the self, with that inflow of breath. The self becomes an extrovert in that inhalation.

17.50. There should be no distinction between the outflow of the breath and the attentive awareness of the intelligence. Both are the same. Using the support of the breath and the *citta* (or mind), with a constant focal point of the very self on the movement of the intelligence and the breath, is known as concrete meditation.

And the state of absolute calm? When both inhalation and exhalation are done without any sort of tension, without any sort of support, it becomes absolute meditation.

17.51. If the inner source of energy is held still and the outflow of breath is allowed to move without tension, the *citta* is silent.

17.52. Can you see my face? Is this a tense brain or not? *Tense*. This is what is taught generally as meditation. Now, again, look at my face: tense brain or not? *Not*. This is how to practice.

This is known as meditation. In this one, the brain is free to move anywhere. In this one the brain cannot think at all, it is caught. So the brain has to do two things: to focus without a focal point. There should be no focal point at all; so the moment you get a focal point, remove it, take it away. The moment it goes means my brain has absolutely no prejudice of any sort; it is completely free by itself.

This is humbleness. I show the humbleness in your brain. As it becomes small, that is humility. The first thing for you to know is if the brain is small or not.

17.53. As you fold your palms in front of your chest, the brain should become humble inside.

17.54. By just bringing the skull down, there is no humility. By releasing the brain from the contact of the skull, there is humility.

17.55. Move the ears deep in, the brain resting on the mind. At the same time, the brain looks at the mind, not allowing the mind to create any vibration in the trunk, and the mind watches the brain, so that the brain is not cut off from the observation, from that humbleness.

17.56. I showed you the tension on my face in that concentration, remember? That tension is known as rigid stillness. So rigid stillness is not a state of silence. The rigidity is a vibration.

17.57. The brain watching the mind and the mind watching the brain, so there is no movement in the brain and the mind. And that is meditation.

17.58. The energy of the brain descending to the seat of the mind, the energy of the mind ascending towards the brain, where they both meet, is the seat of the soul. And there you must live, and that is meditation.

17.59. The movement of inhalation-exhalation is the instrument that has to recognize the Recognizer, the *Atman* inside. So the movement of breath, the organs that you use, the outer ridge of the nostrils, and the lungs have to be completely pure, completely ethical, undisturbed, unwavering.

17.60. As you are inhaling, the unknown, which is called the *Atman*, comes in contact with the known, which is called the mind and the body. In inhalation, the unknown embraces the known, and in exhalation, the known embraces the unknown.

17.61. Exhalation, normal exhalation, should be done in such a way that your brain, your mind, your body, your soul are all completely merged, dissolving into that universal force which is just outside the tip of the nostrils.

17.62. In inhalation, normal inhalation, the cosmic energy is brought in and embraced. In exhalation, the individual energy is drawn out so that it completely mingles or is united with the universal or cosmic energy.

17.63. *During a pranayama class:* Holding is *kumbhaka*. Kumbhaka is not holding the breath, but holding everything in a state of suspense, the suspense of inhalation and of intelligence. Hold the *Atman*, not just the breath.

There is a space between surrender and acceptance. You surrender to the Lord, and the Lord accepts your surrender. And to accept is the state of kumbhaka.

17.64. The Lord which is outside is within. The body which is out should be measured within. What is outside you should be touched inside.

17.65. The brain is the seat of the personality cult. And the mind or intellectual heart is the seat of the impersonality cult.

17.66. Exhalation is the art of surrender.

17.67. It is said that 99 percent perspiration and only 1 percent inspiration is needed. I say yoga pupils need 100 percent perspiration and 100 percent inspiration. So it is with me and you.

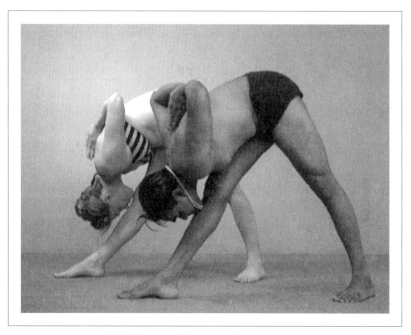

IYENGAR AND NOËLLE IN PARSVOTTANASANA

Not Dated

18.1. Ah! That is the *Om*.

18.2. Yoga is an individual practice but can also be done in society.

18.3. Any holy person is a yogi. Any yogi is a holy person.

18.4. After forty years of age, we live on the energy stored up in youth. There is no more metabolism, just catabolism. We practice yoga to recover. What we do for ourselves is to recover for others; it is sacrifice.

18.5. According to yoga books, yoga is a secret and a sacred subject. I give the secrets to you, but making it sacred is up to you.

18.6. The sun shines everywhere; it does not shine only here and there. In the same way, yoga is for everyone.

18.7. Yoga becomes spiritual when the mind sees what is taking place. If the mind is not seeing, it is physical yoga.

18.8. In yoga, the body disciplines the mind, and the mind disciplines the body. The mind cannot think of the soul as long as it is connected to the body. The body must be trained to be the servant, not the master.

18.9. If someone praises you, you are living in the emotions, not in real life.

18.10. How can you have peace of mind when there is no peace in the body?

18.11. Seeing the intelligence of the body means developing the art of intelligence in observation.

18.12. Sit away from the wall; I may need to kick you.

18.13. Open the golden body with a golden key. You all use your iron brain. Lightness means the brain can see.

18.14. If the lungs collapse, the brain becomes dull, morose.

18.15. You have to get rid of borders, limits, and classifications; then light comes. We see everything on the screen of our ideas. We must get rid of that screen to be able to see what is behind. X's ideas are limited, that is why he remains on the surface. Y got rid of the limits, so she always goes to the depths. We should always meet other people and new subjects with no set frame of mind. We have to live like that even after long acquaintance. We must get rid of every set idea to approach everything and everyone with love.

18.16. In our spiritual quest, we are required to develop our body in such a way that it is no longer a hindrance, but becomes our friend. Similarly, our emotions and intellect must be developed for divine purposes.

18.17. We should see without passion people that we do not love.

18.18. If you open the armpits, the brain becomes light, and you cannot brood or become depressed.

18.19. There is a space between action and silence.

18.20. Circumferential action occurs when the vertical and horizontal meet. If you have to stretch vertically, stretch horizontally as well. When you stretch both ways, the brain is mature.

18.21. The actions of a man mirror his personality better than his words. The yogi has learned the art of dedicating all his actions to the Lord, and so he reflects the Divinity within him.

18.22. Physical balance is opposed to mental balance. Imbalance in a pose is physical yoga. A balanced pose is spiritual yoga.

18.23. If a teacher makes a mistake, all his pupils imitate him. Only a pupil may commit mistakes. Teachers must not commit mistakes. I purge my teachers so they will teach better.

18.24. Nothing comes easily. After hard work, when the *sadhak* has matured, it comes instantaneously, without effort or thought. But the effort cannot be forgotten.

18.25. I am only cross when you do incorrect postures. When you are correct, I am pleased.

18.26. A person who uses the word *hate* is half mad.

18.27. If the throat is passive, the mind is quiet.

18.28. In your asana, use *karma*, *jnana*, and *bhakti* yoga.

18.29. The pupils should challenge the teacher.

18.30. The yoga student should have clarity, faith, devotion, passion, courage.

18.31. Knowing the minimum, you must do your maximum.

18.32. You are all experts—experts at making mistakes.

18.33. Sit in this asana and accept chronological authority. Chronological authority is no authority, as time is just a movement in space.

18.34. Extension brings space, space brings freedom, freedom brings precision. Precision is truth, and truth is God.

18.35. Teach children from the psychological and not the physical point of view alone.

If children do standing poses precisely, head balance comes automatically.

No philosophy. Teach by rotation, by numerals: 1, 2, 3, 4, often jumping from number to number to keep them alert and the mind attentive.

Endurance is not the same with different ages; therefore, have a different syllabus.

Schools do not always have the required equipment, blankets, cleanliness, and so on, so adjust yoga according to the conditions and environment.

No straining, no extension. Only play. No precision in movement; extension and precision only from the age of fifteen.

Don't worry about back bendings; they do those easily enough.

18.36. *Regarding impotency:* Teach asana to activate the nerves. Just doing the pose will not help; one must feel the spasm of life when the contractions take place, where the blood flows.

18.37. We have hospitals to make the sick well again, but do we have anything except yoga to keep the healthy people healthy?

18.38. Why sing *Om*? Om is in your own body.

18.39. Humbleness is the art of learning.

18.40. *Regarding relaxation:* Let the facial skin drop sideways. Let both eyes be equally passive.

18.41. By controlling body intelligence, you control mental intelligence. Physical intelligence is aggressive; mental intelligence is dull. The inside intelligence should penetrate the outside intelligence. Purge the body to purge the brain. The extension of intelligence is pliability. No rigidity is the basis of intelligence.

18.42. The art of relaxation and the art of stretching go together.

18.43. *For sexual frustration:* Find out first if it is physical or mental. It is mostly physical with youngsters, mental with grown-ups. Persons who do not measure their capacity, who go beyond their capacity, wear themselves out through overindulgence.

First, build up strength through head and neck balance, not less than one hour a day, with variations. Then the physical: when the mind demands, is it a physical or mental need?

Give pranayama to create passivity. When the body demands, do the Cobbler's Pose (*Baddha Konasana*) which creates passivity. Stay in the pose not because it brings pleasure, but because of the awareness: "Let me see what it brings."

18.44. Do the maximum, knowing the minimum. Then break your maximum to go further and further.

18.45. If pupils come, say, "Thank God, I have someone to teach." If pupils do not come, say, "Thank God, I am free. I can practice for myself."

18.46. Do your maximum to go further.

18.47. The beginning of humility is to say, "I know nothing, even about the first pose."

18.48. Total action brings total relaxation.

18.49. If the vocal diaphragm is relaxed, the brain is relaxed. There is pain which is visible and pain which is not visible. Hidden pains have to be brought to the surface to be eradicated. Peace of body and poise of mind. As long as there is tightness in body and mind, there is no peace. There are two ways: to live in pain and see if I can eradicate it, or to live with the pain. Internal mistakes create habits.

18.50. Has each part of me done my job correctly?

18.51. All would find their own fruits if they would only listen.

18.52. Profound observation—all points working together.

18.53. Watch carefully between mind and body.

18.54. Follow energy; move with the flow of energy. Do not brake and accelerate together.

18.55. Presence of mind means synchronism between your body and mind.

18.56. Do not do chronological timing without acting psychologically. The brain must work.

18.57. As we take pleasures happily, we should take pains happily when they come. As we live in pleasure, we should learn to see good in pain. Learn to find comfort even in discomfort.

18.58. Everyone comes to yoga to relax.

18.59. You have to get freedom in your body before you can see the spiritual light.

18.60. If the joints are hard, there is a traffic jam in our body. There should be freedom to act.

18.61. Observe the defects of nature, and work against them to convert to a normal state. Then effort ceases.

18.62. Keep intelligence in contact with movement.

18.63. For nonhandicapped people, a crooked body has a crooked brain.

18.64. The brain must see the movement.

18.65. Learn serenity of the body before you learn serenity of the mind. When you struggle, the brain jerks. Presence of body and presence of mind should unite.

18.66. All eight steps of yoga are taught in each posture. There is no division. Total living in *samadhi*.

18.67. Yoga harmonizes body, mind, and soul. It takes away weakness and strengthens the body and mind.

18.68. When there is strain, it is physical yoga. When the brain is passive, it is spiritual yoga.

18.69. *Sutra* means "a thread." As pearls are held on a thread, all the limbs of your body should be held on that thread which is called intelligence.

18.70. Let me act with my soul; let my soul come in communion with the body. That is harmony.

18.71. When the legs are shaky, the mind is also shaky.

18.72. The yogi believes that every creature has as much right to live as he has. He believes that he is born to help others, and he looks upon creation with eyes of love. He knows that his life is linked inextricably with that of others, and he rejoices if he can help them to be happy. He puts the happiness of others before his own and becomes a source of joy to all who meet him. As parents encourage a baby to walk the first steps, he encourages those less fortunate than himself and makes them fit for survival.

18.73. When the body wants to do the asana and you do not want to do it, that is irreligious work.

18.74. If there is no inner light, use the outer light.

18.75. Meditative brain: intelligence everywhere, vastness.

18.76. To understand the world, you open your eyes. To understand the inside world, you should close your eyes.

18.77. During relaxation, when you are intent on stillness, any movement of any sort is a sensual movement. And in any posture, any unconscious, involuntary movement is a sensual movement.

18.78. The eyes are the windows of the brain; the ears are the windows of the soul.

18.79. Your eye should be single: *Atma*.

18.80. Nature is simple; man has made it complicated. We have gone from simplicity to complexity. We should go back to simplicity.

18.81. The candle is fading, so recharge the candle.

18.82. Feeling is the eye.

18.83. Inspiration is the path of creation, and expiration is the path of renunciation.

18.84. Exhale the *jivatman* (individual soul) into the Universal Consciousness.

18.85. In pranayama, the breath is the Lord. Let Him rest in the cradle of the diaphragm, undisturbed.

18.86. An active brain is an aggressive brain. Do not clench your brain as you clench your teeth. Learn to keep the brain receptive while using it.

18.87. Awareness: see behind you before you see inwards.

18.88. You should be aware from moment to moment of what you are doing.

18.89. The art of yoga is beauty in observation.

18.90. Pause between each movement. Then in the stillness, be filled with awareness. Ask yourself, "Has every part of me done its job?" The commander must find out if the soldiers have done their job.

18.91. Be aware of your weakness; that is where you should challenge yourself.

18.92. Uninterrupted intelligence means attention everywhere.

18.93. Do not neglect the poses you can do well. There is always further awareness to develop in the pose.

18.94. If you must cry, cry with great presence of mind.

18.95. *R:* "Guruji, will it be possible for me at my age to learn the new Sun Salutation?"
  Iyengar: "You live within the framework of an idea."
  R: "I want you to confirm that I will be able to do it."
  Iyengar: "You want me to confirm the idea."

18.96. Use fully whatever limited intelligence you have, then automatically it opens a little more and can accumulate more.

18.97. Will over will.

18.98. There is willpower beyond the intellect.

18.99. Patanjali says: Our progress depends on the mild, moderate, or excessive nature of the means employed.

18.100. When the pose is perfect, there is morality.

18.101. Know the morality of each posture. The ethical discipline of the posture is when you are extending correctly and to the maximum.

18.102. The art of stretching is an ethical principle.

18.103. You should become religious within yourself.

18.104. Religion is realization, not denomination. Religion is to remember: know thyself.

18.105. From freedom of the body comes freedom of the mind, and then the Ultimate Freedom.

18.106. A smoker cannot meditate, and a meditator cannot smoke.

18.107. Conscious effort in the back, and visual effort in the front: brain and mind must function as one.

18.108. Patanjali said, Be hard as a diamond and soft as a petal. Intensity alone will build a man.

18.109. I am a teacher for those who have not opened their eyes, but I am a learner still.

18.110. Regarding atrophied muscles, where there is pain, there is life.

18.111. To stick to the truth does not require cleverness. It is only untruth that demands cleverness.

18.112. The meeting of nature and consciousness is a divine marriage. Nature is energy. All the energy of nature should be united with consciousness.

18.113. Stability is a fundamental need in meditation. Emotional stability is necessary for meditation.

18.114. Opening the eyes wide releases pain and stops dullness of the brain.

18.115. Like the waters of the Ganges flowing on the Siva-linga, the exhalation flows inside, on the *linga* that gives life, keeping it neat and pure forever.

18.116. Feel the stretch of the bone, not the flesh. Stretch the skin, then the muscle.

18.117. If you keep aiming at the maximum, Self-knowledge will come. The minimum is sensual yoga. The moment you go a little more than the body can take, you are nearer the Self. The minute you say, "I am satisfied," the light is fading.

18.118. What is required is culture of the heart and hand, not merely culture of the head.

18.119. Truth is very rigid.

18.120. The rays of the sun extend everywhere, but the source remains the same.

18.121. To love is to be merciless.

18.122. In the midst of death, life persists. In the midst of darkness, light persists. In the midst of untruth, truth persists.

18.123. Meditation is not a question to be discussed. Meditation has no frontier, whereas concentration has.

18.124. When the ego is used as an instrument, then the real Self shines.

18.125. If the skin on the skull is hard, this is the result of an artificial meditation. You must create space between the skull and the brain.

18.126. The front brain deals only with the external world. Quieten this brain and retire within. The back brain leads inside. We use only the front brain when we are in distress. Use the back brain for meditation.

18.127. The highest form of surrender is meditation.

18.128. There is something common in each and every one in meditation.

18.129. Truth is one. All experience the same state of mind in meditation: zero state, nonaggressive, not dull. (A dull body gives a dull mind.) Descend the conscious center first.

18.130. Meditation is one of the hardest and finest adjustments of our intellect.

18.131. A swoon is not *samadhi*.

18.132. All three minds are conscious. When the consciousness becomes finer and finer, that is *samadhi*. *Trance* is the wrong word, because it implies an extreme state of consciousness where you forget yourself. To live in the conscious mind is samadhi. You are alive and alone, without a conscious movement.

18.133. Spiritual practice is doing poses well. Convert Hatha Yoga into Raja Yoga by perfecting the poses. What you think of as Raja Yoga is only cultivation of the ego. Use intelligence in action, both factual and analytical. Introversion is meditation.

18.134. Abstract meditation is like an abstract action.

18.135. Has each part of me done my job correctly? This is meditation in action. If you know how to act, the correct movement follows.

18.136. The brain is the thinking center. The mind is the thought center. The state of silence is experienced when the thinking center descends and the thought center ascends at the same time. The thinking center takes one to the future, the thought center takes one to the past, and the silent state keeps one in the present, which is pure.

18.137. The mind is a bottomless pit. Stop trying to fill it, as it cannot be filled. In this way desires will come to an end. Then go beyond that bottomless pit to realize the Self.

18.138. When the brain is still, then meditation begins.

18.139. How can you have *Atma-darsan* (Self-realization) if you cannot surrender the body?

18.140. When you cannot do an exercise, it means the brain has stuck and put up a frontier. Examine the situation closely, and break down the barrier. Meditation has no frontiers.

18.141. Position God for every asana, so you can exert towards Him.

18.142. Each asana should be your God.

18.143. *To a student who wanted to say* japa *while doing postures:* In a posture, japa is the feeling. The feeling is the meaning of action and adjustment.

18.144. Each movement is a mantra; each movement is a God.

18.145. You are only using one arm. Why did God give you two?

18.146. Taking a correspondence course in yoga is like taking a correspondence course with God.

18.147. The spine must never be relaxed, but must reach up to God.

18.148. When things happen without effort, that is the will of the Lord.

18.149. The mind is the outer layer of the Self, and the Self extends everywhere. When you do the pose, you should have that vastness of the mind, not the brain in its place. The brain is only a seat, like your finger.

18.150. Overenthusiasm in teaching is ego.

18.151. What you know, teach well; what you do not know, do not teach. Do not teach until you have attained maturity, or you will not be able to bear the consequences.

18.152. Keep the sympathetic nerves under control, and the parasympathetic nerves are free to work for the soul.

18.153. Balance in space. Go into the unknown. Conquer fear.

18.154. To get freedom, you have to bear pain.

18.155. Without God's will, not even a blade of grass can move.

18.156. When your soul comes before God, He won't ask, "What did you do first?" He will say, "What did you do last?"

18.157. They worship their teacher when he tells them to do head balance with their eyes closed. How can they see God?

18.158. I have shown you all a glimpse of eternity.

18.159. *L:* "During meditation, I got pins and needles in my feet, and all my concentration was on my feet."
   Iyengar: "That was also a good meditation."

18.160. Truth is the experienced understanding of the unity of the cognizer and the cognized. In the moment of truth, there is silence in the awareness of oneness.

18.161. Truth is dynamic and uncompromising.

18.162. Only fact is the truth.

18.163. Without experiencing human love and happiness, it is not possible to know Divine love.

18.164. How many languages do I speak? Only one, the language of love.

18.165. Geometrical adjustment: you must be balanced. Use both sides of the mind.

18.166. If you use violence to balance, how can you convert it to non-violence?

18.167. Contraction brings tension to the nerves; release brings freedom.

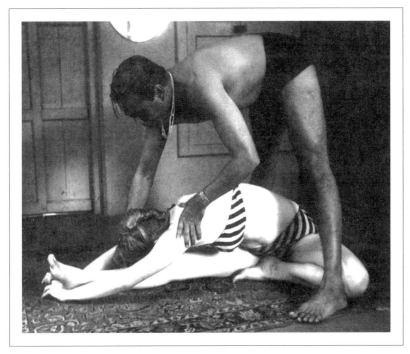

IYENGAR WITH NOËLLE IN JANU SIRSASANA

18.168. Whatever is nearest the ground, that portion is the brain for understanding the posture.

18.169. If you are stretching the right leg, the left leg should not collapse.

18.170. There is a dual personality in the brain.

18.171. Horizontal extension and vertical extension should synchronize together.

18.172. The front part of the brain deals with the outside world; the back part deals with the internal world and is for the study of the Self.

18.173. Failure in the cultivation of the Self is due to intoxicated intelligence. If my intelligence is superior to yours, you must use that superior intelligence. We are all intoxicated with our own confusion.

18.174. It is the Self that acts, not the intelligence.

18.175. The ocean is the Self; the waves are the thoughts. The Self is silent in the same way as the ocean is silent—the waves make the noise.

18.176. Purge the self; do not be contented.

18.177. As long as you do not live totally in the body, you do not live totally in the Self. Total awareness.

18.178. The body is inert: *tamas*. The mind is active: *rajas*. The Self is pure: *sattva*. The body has to be brought up to the lightness of the Self.

18.179. When you give an involuntary groan, it is the sound of the body. When you know the sound of the body, then you know the sound of the soul.

18.180. With perception comes self-correction.

18.181. The asana is an enquiry: "Who am I?" Throwing out the parts until only the Self is left. The final pose is "I am."

18.182. If the mind does not see, it is a small mind. If you cannot see your little toe, how can you see the Self?

18.183. *On Self-realization:* The Self must exist in every pore of the skin.

18.184. Unless you feel the movement of the skin, you do not have sensibility.

18.185. The skin is the sense of knowledge.

18.186. If you cannot see the gross body, you cannot see the Self.

18.187. The soul must work, not the body.

18.188. Without art there is no science. A philosopher is always an artist, and vice versa. Our body is the instrument for our art.

18.189. When you have conquered the microcosm, you have conquered the macrocosm.

18.190. V speaks philosophy all day long, but this philosophy she does not know—the philosophy of her own body.

18.191. If the body collapses, you have to recreate energy.

18.192. In yoga, no limb of the body is kept idle.

18.193. Do not let the physical body drag along.

18.194. The brain is the heaviest limb in our body.

18.195. Become detached from the body.

18.196. *During an explanation of how trees are pruned:* I prune human nature.

18.197. The body is first treated as physical, then the body is used for the discipline of the intellect. By creating intelligence in the body, you refine the intellect.

18.198. Do not contract your brain when you stretch your body.

18.199. Where was the man when he jumped off the bridge?
  "On the bridge?"
  "No, that was before he jumped."
  "In the air?"
  "No, that was after he jumped."
  "In his skin!"

18.200. If you know the extension of the body, you know the extension of the mind. If there is nervousness in the body, the brain has contracted.

18.201. Listen to the sound of the body when it is acting. The body is the dictator of the mind.

18.202. As beginners, our intellect is only in the brain. You must have a million eyes, all over the body.

18.203. Work where it is not functioning. See where it is not moving. Any hardness in the body should be made soft.

18.204. When there is no duality, there is purity. If the front brain is active: duality. If the front brain is passive: purity.

18.205. Comfort comes in the pose only when effort ceases, as after long, persistent practice.

18.206. Not intoxication, but evolution. Intoxication with knowledge is ego culture.

18.207. If the body can do more and you do not do it, it is immoral yoga.

18.208. When there is softness and lightness in the body, the pose is correct; when hardness and heaviness, the pose is wrong. Lightness and softness is total stretch, which means total awareness.

18.209. Total awareness of the body brings total awareness of the self, and total awareness is Raja Yoga.

18.210. Overenthusiasm must be killed, because it is short-lived.

18.211. You have no body realization, yet you want God realization. Experience everything in life, but retain only the good. Divide the body into millions of parts and then stretch; do not attempt to stretch a lump. At that moment only, you are in a state of Divinity: the mind going beyond the known into the unknown. When you feel you have attained the maximum stretch, go beyond. Going beyond the mind is the state of purity. The known is what you consider your maximum. Go beyond, then spiritual practice starts.

18.212. The teacher has to die for the sake of the pupils.

18.213. You should be concerned to be unconcerned.

18.214. To create harmony, work from your heart, not your brain.

18.215. The mind extends vertically into the past, the brain into the future, while the action of the present extends horizontally. So present concentration becomes a holy cross.

18.216. Do not live in the future; only the present is real.

18.217. What I was is unimportant. What I am is important.

18.218. When the pose is correct, there is lightness, freedom. When it is heavy, it is wrong.

18.219. The highest form of sensitivity is the highest form of activity of the intellect.

18.220. The brain should be completely quiet, and the body active.

18.221. To be pure is to act well.

18.222. For a wrong done by others, men demand justice, while for that done by themselves, they plead for mercy and forgiveness. The yogi, on the other hand, believes that for a wrong done by himself there should be justice, while for that done by another there should be forgiveness. He knows and teaches others how to live. Always striving to perfect himself, he shows them by his love and compassion how to improve themselves.

18.223. To be dull is easy. To be active requires tremendous work.

18.224. To live within yourself is to cultivate yourself.

18.225. The still waters of a lake reflect the beauty around it. When the mind is still, the beauty of the Self is reflected in it.

18.226. The brain takes you to the future; the mind takes you to the past; the Self takes you to the present. Past, present, and future are held in each pose. The present is the perfect pose.

When you open horizontally, the future and the past meet in the present. Vertical ascending is the future; vertical descending is the past. The horizontal is the present.

18.227. A cunning body: a body that is a treacherous friend.

18.228. You cannot jump across a chasm in two jumps.

18.229. Wherever there is a dent in the body, there is no intelligence.

18.230. There should be constant analysis throughout the action, not afterwards. This is understanding. The real meaning of knowledge is that your action and your analysis synchronize.

18.231. A stable brain without laziness: when the intellect is stable there is no past, no future, only the present.

18.232. We must be bold; we must be cautious.

18.233. You all want to act with the intelligence of the brain, not the intelligence of the heart.

18.234. There must be mobility of the intellect to get stability of the body.

18.235. Learning can be acquired, but wisdom must be earned.

18.236. Limited knowledge will give you a limited approach. Unlimited knowledge has an unlimited source.

18.237. No challenge, no response. Both should be equal at the time of action. No future without a perfect present. If the present is correct or rightly done, the future takes care of itself. The challenge and the response to challenge must be the same. Then precision in action comes. If there is a disparity or difference, then the action does not become perfect, as the clarity of the intelligence gets clouded.

18.238. An introvert will appear to be listening to every word but will not have taken in a thing.

18.239. The mind should not sleep. Create mobility.

18.240. Every right action contains its own propaganda.

18.241. There should be harmony in action. See and act.

18.242. Humility in action.

18.243. Analyze in action, not intellectually and objectively (without movement).

18.244. If you know how to act, correct movement follows.

18.245. Stupidity and sincerity cannot go together. Only sincerity and intelligence can go together.

18.246. Descending intelligence is faster than ascending intelligence.

18.247. When I took my daughter Geeta off medicine and made her do asana, the doctor said, "There is an improvement; continue the medicine."

18.248. Did you have an experience of marriage before marriage? No! Will you try head balance before head balance?

18.249. You must not seek, you must search. You must not see, you must look at. You must not hear, you must listen to. You must not touch, you must palpate. You must not smell, you must sniff.

18.250. When a posture is accurate or defective, observe what is the state of the intellect.

18.251. Use your mind as a mirror to adjust yourself. Has my mind imprinted the correct movement or not?

18.252. Either I will break your back, or you will break mine. I don't know which of us will go to heaven first. Perhaps it will be you. You are all selfish people.

18.253. Relaxation follows extension. We cannot maintain continuity of intensity. That we have to learn.

18.254. Create awareness in your pupils.

18.255. The young, the old, the extremely aged, even the sick and the infirm obtain perfection in yoga by constant practice. Success will follow him who practices, not him who practices not. Success in yoga is not obtained by the mere theoretical reading of sacred texts. Success is not obtained by wearing the dress of a yogi or a *sannyasin*, nor by talking about it. Constant practice alone is the secret of success. Verily, there is no doubt about this.

18.256. Anything treated casually does not bear rich fruit. Doing things casually is not religious minded.

18.257. The madman shouts out loud. The average human intellectual calculates within. The wise man does not speak internally or externally, but remains silent within and without.

18.258. A passive neck goes with activity and right action.

18.259. Learn to find passivity in activity.

18.260. Charity is not cleverness. It is a virtue by itself.

18.261. Profound observation is a must at all moments of action.

18.262. Do to your capacity. Always strive to extend your capacity. Ten minutes today, after a few days, twelve minutes. Master that, then again extend.

18.263. Fright should descend; confidence should ascend.

18.264. Karma Yoga is skill in action.

18.265. While doing yoga, your body must tell you what to do, not your brain.

18.266. There is dull action, and there is intelligent action.

18.267. Analyze in action, not intellectually without action.

18.268. We behave as though we know more than we actually know.

18.269. Watch your base; be attentive to the portion nearest the floor.

18.270. The character of precision is to bear pain in order to reach the ultimate. Every soul has a goal in life, that is, to reach God. When the soul reaches its goal, both lose their identities. That is God or the Divine.

18.271. Experience what death is: look with the internal eye, the conscious eye.

18.272. Walk into a class; don't show off.

18.273. Bring all efforts to their fullness to awaken *kundalini*.

18.274. Give pupils complete action and then complete relaxation. Total action brings total relaxation. Do yoga fully well, and relax at the end.

8.275. Teacher and thought must be in communion.

18.276. No challenge, no response, so no pure action. The response must be as strong as the challenge; to realize awareness, the response must be felt.

18.277. Do not move the whole body to adjust a particular movement in the body.

18.278. To implant an idea in a person's mind is often an obstacle and not a help.

18.279. To stop yawning, inhale and hold the breath. Introverts yawn more; they are not in communion.

18.280. Chronological time and psychological time are quite different.

18.281. Not one pose comes with ease.

18.282. A dull part is a sign of weakness in that area.

18.283. Exhale with the movement.

18.284. *To E, who has liver trouble:* Think liver, that my liver is my philosophy. Concentrate on the liver; that is meditation. The liver teaches you philosophy.

18.285. Convert from the external to the internal.

18.286. Nobody can go to heaven unless the foundation is firm.

18.287. *R said:* I heard a fellow squealing out for mercy as he strained, and I thought I knew the voice, and it was me!

18.288. Some turn ugliness into beauty, and some turn beauty into ugliness.

18.289. The third eye is the thought center, which must be transcended.

18.290. My blood oozes inwards when I see movement (and not action).

18.291. Excitement goes with action. Never be excited by movement.

18.292. The thought center, *manas chakra* (*citta stana*), must be transcended. I want action, not motion.

18.293. Action is required, not motion.

18.294. *Regarding sitting pose:* Surrender the spine to the floor.

18.295. To keep the brain alert, the spine has to keep the brain in position.

18.296. Be a free man. Inquire, "What am I doing? Why am I doing it? What is happening to me?" That is how to get awareness.

18.297. As you have taken pains to learn, continue with devotion what you have learned.

18.298. If you don't know the source of the action, the action is impure.

18.299. Try all possible ways. The man who says, "I cannot do it" is an escapist and has no religion. To say, "I am better" is escapism—it is the mind making an excuse to stop.

18.300. Yoga is a culture, not a religion. The practice of yoga makes a better Christian.

18.301. If you are good at your yoga, it is immoral not to teach. On the other hand, it is immoral to teach if you are not practicing well yourself.

18.302. When you teach, you are an extrovert. When you learn, you are an introvert.

18.303. If you teach what you do not know, you will bear the consequences.

18.304. Have you completely known the known (the body) before trying to know the Unknown (God)?

18.305. Man has been given the intelligence to distinguish between the sensual and the spiritual. This power of discrimination belongs to man only, not to the animal.

18.306. You must have millions of eyes watching the body.

18.307. You use only the two physical eyes; that is why you are useless.

18.308. *When asked about virility:* A practical defect requires a practical remedy.

18.309. Smoking makes the brain dull. It is only an escape from facing the truth.

18.310. We waste our energy in motion and leave none for action. Action is not motion. Only action can liberate.

18.311. After acting, reflect on what you have done. Has the brain interpreted the action correctly? If the brain does not receive, there is confused action. The duty of the brain is to receive and act. Pause between each movement. The self has to find out whether this has been done well or not.

18.312. There must be relaxation in full extension.

18.313. Earnestness in effort is *tapas*.

18.314. Without clarity, there is no courage.

18.315. Attainment comes when the body has been conquered, not forgotten.

18.316. Diabetes is an emotional disease. The diabetic has first to learn to live with peace of mind.

18.317. Intelligence merges with the flow of energy; no ego.

18.318. When you have intelligence, you need maturity.

18.319. The hardest road is the surest and the shortest one.

18.320. When you challenge the weak part, you must immediately counterchallenge.

18.321. How can you expect fruit from an uncared-for tree?

18.322. Challenge and counterchallenge should weigh evenly on both the left and right sides. Only then will lightness come.

18.323. Hard work without humility is not a spiritual *sadhana*.

18.324. *When someone called him "Iron Iyengar":* I am not hard like iron, but hard like a diamond.

18.325. Philosophy is not a language but the science of language, the study of which will enable the student to learn his own language better. Similarly, yoga is not a religion in itself. It is the science of religion, the study of which will enable a *sadhaka* the better to appreciate his own faith.

18.326. *Swamiji, on observing that L was wearing orange sandals:* "Why do you wear the holy color on your feet?"

L to Iyengar: "What must I answer him?"

Iyengar: "Tell him it is on the top of your feet and not on the bottom."

Swamiji to L: "The light of yoga shines from your eyes."

18.327. *Avidya*, ignorance, has no discipline. When you realize that you are ignorant, discipline begins.

18.328. Learn the "brain" of body movements; there is a very small movement from the source.

18.329. Mistakes can be seen only in a dull body.

18.330. When the brain is silent, it is nonviolent yoga. When the brain is tight, it is violent yoga. The body should be violent and the brain nonviolent.

18.331. I have given you everything, everything. My heart is empty. I have no guilty conscience. I am free. I am giving you all of me—take it.

18.332. I am only violent when the body does not obey.

18.333. Before asking the class to attempt a strenuous pose, tell them a story to make them laugh and relax the body.

18.334. Let us be ripe within ourselves, before we give to others.

18.335. Why would it be a struggle for me to teach? It is my dedication.

18.336. You don't even know how to know if I am a good teacher.

18.337. *N said:* You cannot cheat Iyengar. In the same way that we have to have a million eyes to watch our own body, he has a million eyes to watch us.

18.338. Relax the part where I hit you. If you say you are trying, you are not trying; it is only a mental movement. Don't try, do it.

18.339. Casual people should be treated casually. Dedicated ones, treat with dedication. A casual approach is illusory. Test your pupils. Know the capacity of your pupils.

18.340. If you have done it to please me, you have not done it.

18.341. Give your pupils help because they have no perception.

18.342. The teacher must move with the student.

18.343. The job of the master is to create disappointment to teach humility or there can be no progress.

18.344. A teacher must never express pliability outside, only inside. That is the way to keep pupils alert: no softness in the teacher while teaching.

18.345. If people come to me as teachers and not as pupils, then I create fear in them, which they must conquer. Humbleness is the art of learning.

18.346. It is better to train one pupil honestly than to train thousands.

18.347. Create the pupil's mistakes in your own body, and then do the pose to get the feeling of the wrong movement.

18.348. Humble inside, strong outside.

18.349. I kill your vanity with my vanity.

18.350. The master is one who knows how to come down to the level of the pupil and who knows how to go up.

18.351. The pupil also teaches the master. Looking at the pupil guides the teacher.

18.352. Teach by example.

18.353. A preacher is not a teacher; a preacher is a propagandist.

18.354. Let others teach impurity. Why should I teach what is not pure?

18.355. The art of teaching is tolerance.

18.356. It is easy to attain, but difficult to maintain.

18.357. I don't need to see your teaching. I just have to see the stability and the character of the teacher.

18.358. There is no envy amongst my pupils; they are like one family.

18.359. I give much more than I take. All my teachers have to do the same. They also give far more than they take. Only I may criticize my teachers; no one else has the right to criticize.

18.360. When I teach, I attach myself to my pupils, for that is the only way they can learn. When I have finished, I detach myself. You are free to go. You have done a good job.

18.361. For yourself, be a pessimist inside, an optimist outside. Positivity works on negativity. We must be 90 percent desperate and only 10 percent hopeful.

18.362. These postures are meant to make known the unknown; the unknown has to be brought to the surface.

18.363. Yoga has been given for stability only.

18.364. The third eye is above the middle of the eyebrow, at *lalata chakra*, the center that must be transcended.

The Early Life of B.K.S. Iyengar

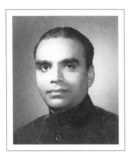

BELLUR IS A SMALL VILLAGE in the Kolar District of the South Indian state of Karnataka. The man who would become Iyengar's father was born there of Brahmin caste. He was given the name of Krishnamachar. He spent part of his life teaching children at the elementary school in the village of Narasapuk Taluk, three kilometers from Bellur. After thirty years of service, he left for Bangalore to work for a wholesaler whom Iyengar says was a Muslim. At that time there was no religious strife in India but great tolerance for any expression of faith.

Krishnamachar married Sheshamma, a very young, simple, and religious woman. Iyengar remembers her as a wonderful mother. He told me that when she visited him in Pune she refused to bathe with water from the faucet; it was to her less pure than well water.

Like many Indians, she was good to everyone. A kind of human solidarity exists in Indian village tradition. The same is still true in rural France, where a visitor could be Jesus disguised as a pilgrim or a beggar and would not be refused bread for fear of refusing God. The same spirit rules in India, the favorite country of the mendicant God-seeker. People don't want to refuse anything for fear of refusing a true saint!

This harmonious couple produced thirteen children. Their father adored them. None of the children remembers having been scolded by this gentle man.

Sundararaja, our Iyengar, was born on Saturday, December 14, 1918, at 3:00 a.m. He was the eleventh child. He was born in the middle of a flu epidemic. His mother was a victim and for a long time their lives were in danger. Thanks to God both survived, but the little Sundararaja remained sickly.

Later, Krishnamachar had the premonition that he would "slip into universal consciousness" when his son reached the age of nine, which is what happened. Extremely difficult years began for the widow and her youngest children. The older ones were already married and with children of their own; they could barely help. During that time, Iyengar really knew hunger and a desperation that drives you to do anything to get food and to get an education. "Desperation and even thoughts of suicide," he admitted.

Krishnamachar had predicted that his son would triumph after many difficult years and that he would raise and support a family, even become famous. This prediction often helped Iyengar and kept him from losing hope.

Iyengar felt a deep affection for his father. In the 1960s, he used his first savings for the construction of an elementary school in Bellur.

One day he told me: "I was not born into a family of saints. I was not destined to practice yoga." But his grandfather, the great Sanskrit specialist Shri Shrinavasa Iyengar, was to go from Mysore to Gujarat, in northern India, to spread the philosophy and faith of Shri Vaishnava. Iyengar brought up all his children in this faith.

The Origin of His Name

Iyengar has a family name preceded by three first names or initials, which is contrary to southern village tradition. Why?

Social integration in lineage and locality is very strong in India. A man is given a first name that will be preceded by the initials of his father and his village. Following that system, Iyengar would be called B.K. Sundararaja. Where does the name by which he is known, Iyengar, come from? When Yehudi Menuhin took him to Europe in 1954, he needed a passport, and it required a family name. He put down the name of the large family group he was a member of—his clan, you could say—a name made famous by many holy men and philosophers. Since then he has always kept this name.

To get this precious passport, he also needed a certificate to prove that he had paid all his taxes, so he had to pay! "I am probably the only yogin who paid any," he said with a laugh.

An Ordinary Man

Paying taxes did not bother Iyengar. He wanted to be a common man like anyone else, one who fits well into society. The temptation to play the *sannyasin*, or holy man, never crossed his mind. He never had the idea to single himself out with the fashions and customs of his country, as do so many Indians coming to Europe or the United States. For him, that is folklore and has nothing to do with true spiritual development, true sainthood. It has nothing to do with *artha* (purpose) or with *dharma* (virtue).

As an orthodox Brahmin, he respected all the rules of his cast and his community, so that his children would have the opportunity to get married and be happy. He says that action should be guided by intelligence and love, which motivated the rules originally, but they have become more restrictive over time. However, he has adjusted himself to this rigid frame. This is artha.

For example, a Brahmin cannot touch the untouchables or a Westerner. However, he always touched us, and he has always touched the untouchables. "They are men as we are," he said.

And when he noticed that Western men don't wear their hair long, he cut his Brahmin hair-bun in 1954.

The Cow

In India the cow is revered religiously, as it was by the Aryan cowherds thousands of years ago. This sacred cult of the cow was kept alive throughout history, despite the influence of the various invaders of the highly civilized Dravidian fertile valleys.

Iyengar demonstrated this belief one day in Switzerland when we passed a stable. He opened the door saying, "Let me pay my respects to my Goddess," and proceeded to caress their beautiful rumps. "How beautiful they are and well fed. Remember our cows? How happy they would be here!" In his gesture was the same respect and tenderness shown by people who caress the foot of a statue of St. Peter or a miraculous Virgin.

Touch is a profound gesture to an Indian. Touch of the hand or forehead, any contact as an exchange between two people, is felt strongly in India, where nobody touches in greeting.

Courage, Humor, and Modesty

Iyengar is a courageous man, not put off by difficulties, unstoppable in his tireless effort. Every year he continues to make progress, finding a purer, more beautiful way to approach an asana, going further into the details of perfecting a pose. Stagnation is death, he likes to say, but then adds gently that "at your stage effort dominates, at mine it is zeal." Zeal is passion, and passion does not mean it is easy or there is no suffering! Zeal stimulates you to work continuously without dislike or boredom, but it pushes you also to continue beyond what you know. He says that what is known is in the bag; what is interesting is beyond and still unknown.

He always has a joke ready, a great, infectious smile, sarcasm and humor to soften the cracking of the whip. Working hard with him is not funny, but it is never tragic. In the end, there is always mildness or a practical joke.

When he was young, he wanted to know if he was on the right path, and every time he met a yogin, he proposed a mutual exchange or collaboration. An old yogi told him one day: "You do as much as the *rishi* of the Himalayas," and that really encouraged him to continue.

Always this same affirmation came when he met a sage, a saint, or a yogin, be it Swami Sivananda, Vibhatijoti Swami, or Swami Ramananda, who was so holy that he was buried and not cremated. He met these swamis around 1940.

A very old yogin said something that struck him. "How does a tree know that it gives shade and that the shade is good? How can you know at what level you are? Continue." And he went on. You could say that his life is an incessant effort towards perfection.

Powers

In 1959 he spoke to me of *siddhis*, what we call powers. When you realize that you have a power, you must be happy that you made progress, but don't use it, he warned. He gave me an example. "In Bombay a student always asked me to give him a number. I did not understand why, but to please him I said the first number that popped in my head. Then another student on another day asked me the same thing and I refused, smiling. I wasn't going to waste class time to give numbers! But the second student got upset and said, "Why did you give it to him and not to me?" Then I learned from him that the number I gave was always the winning number at the races. I stopped giving numbers immediately. I was not even tempted to use it for myself."

Iyengar gave another example of a man who used his powers to make money. His spiritual development stopped, and he became crippled.

When you read his writings or hear him speaking about powers, you get the impression that they are something to be lived with. They arrive despite you. They are not something pleasant to be looked for, for satisfaction or glory. If we work honestly and in depth, it is just a sign from heaven confirming that we are on the right way.

He used to say humbly: "I am on the path. How can one say that one has arrived?" And he would add that you must not read, but experience. "I read only when something new happens to me; then I look for what Patanjali says about it."

The Gift of Intuition

Several times he surprised me, telling me what I had done the evening before and where I was going to go that afternoon. One day I arrived in Pune for my class and told him that I would go to the horse races in the afternoon. He said, "I know, an hour ago I was thinking that you were going to go there." Exactly one hour before, my friend Mani had called to invite me.

In 1960 in Gstaad during a lesson: "You went to Mount Eggli yesterday, I saw you there." It was true, but how could he have seen me? I kept asking him questions to solve this puzzle. He had fun; it was like a game for him. Finally I asked how I was dressed. "The same as today," he laughed. He was wrong. Finally I had the solution: he had not seen me with his eyes.

In 1959 he told me: "You will write books." We were in the little room where we worked. The sun made a great rectangle on the floor, so it was late September, at the end of the monsoon. I was surprised: "Me? But Sir, I don't know anything!" He insisted: "Today you don't, but one day you will have a lot to say and you will write. Believe me."

A Sense of Devotion

He said, "I am a teacher to those who still have their eyes closed, but I always remain a student." Such words convey the humble attitude of all great searchers, be they saints or scientists.

Devotion is another quality of the master, who never complains and keeps a positive attitude. "When you get students, thank God that you have someone to teach. When no one shows up, thank God for being free to work more on yourself."

He wrote me one day, "When the Lord wants us to dedicate more time to our own work, He Himself will provide. If he does not provide, we have to work and praise Him continuously."

Ramamani, Protecting Angel and Beloved Spouse

Ramamani was born November 2, 1927. I don't think I exaggerate when I say that Iyengar is where he is today thanks to her. It is true that he himself is courageous, intelligent, and ardent in his pursuits, but his evolution has been greatly supported by the loving atmosphere she created around him. She left us on January 28, 1973.

They had a wonderful marriage. It began in complete poverty, as Iyengar said, "with only a *sari* and a *dhoti*." I have rarely seen two people love each other as much and in every way. The hardships of his youth and his sensitive nature had taught Iyengar many things. He explained one day: "In marriage the key to a happy life is sensual pleasure. I satisfied my wife, and we lived in peace and happiness." What a wonderful husband he must have been!

One day in 1960 in Brussels, when he had come to give some lessons to his "dear queen," queen Elisabeth of Belgium, we walked around looking for the famous statue of Manneken Pis. Iyengar gaily made lighthearted jokes about the ways he could give a souvenir of the statue to his wife, and we laughed like two silly kids!

We spoke a lot about her and about happy couples and he said, "Today I am going to write my wife that to live in a palace without you gives me no pleasure. What good is a big bed and all this splendor when you are not by my side?" In fact, he was staying in a very nice room at Palace Stuyvenberg, where the queen lived. Iyengar was very comfortable there. He is comfortable anywhere, with the greats of the world and with the little people, in a palace or in a shantytown.

In my eyes, Ramamani was the incarnation of the perfect spouse: unassuming when he was there and perfect head of family in his absence. Such "spiritual gymnastics" always fascinated me. One day Savita got very sick and emitted a nauseating odor. Her mother really wanted to call the doctor, but Iyengar was against it. "Let me think about it," he said. The fever rose, but Ramamani did not get the doctor. When the fever rose still higher, she insisted again, but in respect for her husband she waited for his permission. Then Iyengar had a brilliant idea: he closed one of Savita's nostrils and told her to blow very hard, and then repeated it on the other side. Finally a hard piece of petrified blood came out. It reeked; they had to open the windows. But the child was cured.

Iyengar adored his wife. The first thing he would do after arriving in Gstaad was to pick me up: "Come and help me pick out a ring for my wife."

The ring was put on hold and paid off gradually as he received money from his lessons.

In Pune he was in the habit of coming down to Bombay every Saturday to teach a class at the end of the afternoon. Sunday mornings he would give another one and then take the train back around noon to arrive in Pune in early evening. One day I asked him, "Does it not bother your wife to spend every weekend without you?"

"No, why?"

"She might like to be with you."

"My wife does not think like that; if she did, I would not do it." What a sweet answer! This woman's heart was pure love. And Iyengar's was as well.

Separation

When Iyengar found himself alone after the death of his wife, he had this comment: "All these years I was a *sannyasin* with a wife. Now I am a house-holder without a wife!" Iyengar can only be described as a paradox; he seems to be pulled between extremes. It shows a dimension of his rich personality.

He had not foreseen this heartbreaking separation, which came so quickly. His plan was different: "When we have married off all our children, I will leave for the Himalayas with my wife. In general, men go alone. But I do not want to abandon her. She has given me everything; she has sacrificed for me. I will take her with me." And as usual he added, "If God bless us." God judged otherwise.

Did she help this man she loved so much "from above"? No one will ever know, and Iyengar keeps his secrets. But when I saw him again after the death of his wife, he had bounced back, as far as I could judge. In response to a letter in which I had carefully tried to pose some subtle questions, he answered: "Where I arrived I don't know, but I do know that God has given me in yoga beyond my capacities." In another letter, he wrote: "The yoga that helped me enjoy myself fully and legitimately with my wife, this same yoga led me to an inner depth at the moment when the Lord in his kindness called my wife to Him. He took my wife away for me to practice yoga all alone."

The Children

Iyengar says that he has had six daughters and one son. Geeta, the oldest, was born December 7, 1944. When I was in India, she was fourteen years old and already wore a little sari. In 1959 Iyengar would accept her often into the yoga class with me, to encourage her. For me it was a joy to see this willowy vine, full of courage and eagerness. She made such quick progress, really had it in her blood! But don't think that Iyengar was softer on his daughter than he was with us; he was an even more demanding guru to her. Geeta chose to remain single to be completely dedicated to her art. In this way, the second daughter, Vanita, could be married. She was born August 29, 1947.

"My next daughter died after the delivery," says Iyengar. "I dreamed that I would lose this child. I wrote my wife, who was then in Bangalore, and it was exactly what had happened."

One day Iyengar said to his wife: "Last night I came to you, and you shall deliver a son." It makes you think of the biblical patriarchs. Sure enough, the fourth child was a son. He came into the world July 2, 1949. "During the night I dreamed of Mahatma Gandhi, and he blessed me. I don't remember the day exactly, but the next morning I told my wife that we were going to have a son. For that reason, I called him Prashant: Peace. He is peaceful and likes philosophy."

Everything went well, until one day Prashant was found dead. Iyengar demonstrated with arms together, palms up, how he had carried him to the cremation field.

"Did you cry?"

"No, why? I prayed."

When they got to the cremation field, the little boy came to life and opened his eyes. No one ever could explain what happened.

"He is an odd child," Iyengar told me in 1959. "He does not want to speak to women, except for his mother and sisters. You will see; he will not speak to you. He is there, looks at you, but will not speak with you. I think that he will be a great philosopher."

Prashant received his Brahmanic cord in the ceremony of Brahmopa-desham on February 7, 1960, during a waxing moon. He loves music, and he took up the violin due to the friendship with Menuhin. He plays it Indian style. Later he applied himself to yoga and now helps his father with the institute.

The girls are all pretty, one as much as the other. After Vanita came Sunita and then Suchita, born July 3, 1951, and July 21, 1953, respectively.

And finally Savita arrived. She was four years old when I knew her (her birthdate is May 5, 1955). She was a little, dark brown thing with enormous black eyes, a lively little savage that I tried to tame for two and a half months. When I arrived, she scampered off proclaiming to anyone who wanted to hear, "The girl that's bigger than a house has arrived!"

One day during my lesson, she was in the little room. She was very good; nobody heard her. Iyengar had placed me in Sarvangasana, and without being able to see, I felt a finger sliding over the skin of my back. Iyengar often gives instructions this way—you obey his finger or his eye—so I stretched. Again, a sliding of the fingers: I stretched more, or at least tried to, because I was already at my limit. And again.

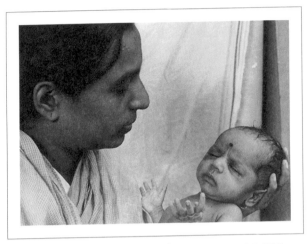
SAVITA IYENGAR WITH IYENGAR'S FIRST GRANDSON, 1973

"I cannot do more, Sir. I really don't understand what you are asking of me," I said.

"But I did not say anything," answered Iyengar.

"But who is touching me then?"

Well, it was Savita, who passed her little finger over my back, then over the skin on her arm, and so on, to see if there was a difference between my skin and hers. You can imagine how we all had a good laugh over that.

Savita is now twenty years old (in 1975) and dances the Bharata Natyam, the dance of South India. She applies herself with the same zeal that her father stimulates in everyone who approaches him.

Iyengar is an exceptional father, tender and firm. All his children adore him. The year his wife died, he came to give his usual seminars in Europe and the U.S. But he would go back to Pune every month—one month gone, one month at home. "I must be both father and mother and get them slowly used to being without me," he explained.

In 1959 I was the only foreign student and had the extraordinary opportunity to enter into the intimacy of this marvelous family.

Iyengar's Guru

A guru is extremely important in the life of someone who wants to advance seriously in a certain discipline. It is the image of the elder who takes you by the hand, the image of God, even. For the fake gurus of India or Europe, the temptation is great to give in to the adoration of students who have become their followers. Those followers like to create a cult, blinded by a personality who deceives them and may elevate himself to the level of deity. There are plenty of those in India. Sadly, the same is true in France.

This was not the case with Shri Krishnamacharya, Iyengar's guru, who was extremely severe and did not tolerate this little game. Iyengar revered Krishnamacharya with enduring love and respect that never diminished, despite the sometimes harsh treatment by the guru.

The first time Iyengar spoke about him to me was in 1959 in Pune. He said: "My guru is my brother-in-law, the husband of my oldest sister. He came to see my mother one day and I was coughing. My mother was widowed, and we depended on people willing to help us. This was in 1934. He came up to Bombay for a tour of yoga demonstrations. Bangalore, where we lived, was on his way. He asked if I wouldn't go and stay with my sister while he was gone. And that is how I joined the *yogasala* of Mysore that he directed. When he came back, he asked me to stay and taught me some poses."

Hanumanasana

Iyengar tells this story about an incident that happened with his teacher. "One day a visitor came and asked the Guruji for instructions about

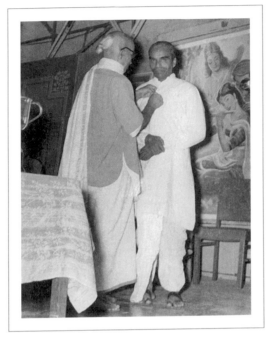

Hanumanasana (the great split); he did not understand how to do it. Guruji had me do the pose. I was very stiff and still very new, and I thought that he did not remember the difficulty I had with this pose. But how could I remind him? I only spoke one language, and it was the same one spoken by the visitor. So I said that I could not do it because my shorts were too tight. Guruji asked one of his students to get a pair of scissors in the kitchen and cut open the seams of my shorts; then he told me to do the pose. Because I did not want to put my brother-in-law to shame, I did the best I could and more, forcing a lot. For months afterward I suffered with a pulled thigh muscle. Because of the fear he inspired, I could never tell him. This taught me that you had to go far, but without forcing. Brutality is not the same as giving of yourself."

Departure for Pune

Iyengar continued: "In 1936 Guruji left with several students to make a tour of yoga demonstrations. I was one of the students. A surgeon by the name of Dr. V.B. Gokhale was very impressed by our demonstration. Later, when this Dr. Gokhale retired and settled in Pune, he wrote Guruji, requesting him to send a man to Pune to teach yoga for six months. I already had given many demonstrations, but Guruji would have preferred to send an older and more experienced student. Everyone he asked refused. Finally he turned to me and said: 'Do you want to go?' I answered: 'I will do what you tell me,' and he told me to go.

"I have to admit that I was happy with this offer, which allowed me freedom and escape from the fear that my guru inspired. It was only for six months; it was worth a try.

"It was very hard: I left everything I knew. I left for the north of Deccan, a town where no one spoke my language and I did not speak theirs. The customs are very different there from those in the true south, where I come from.

"To earn the price of my train ticket to Pune, I walked 22 kilometers every day during one month, from Dhawar to Habli, to give a lesson.

"I really put up with a lot: I arrived in Pune with simply a dhoti and a shirt and one rupee in my pocket. It was 1937. I already told you that God did not bless me until after I passed a test: at the place where I was teaching, someone burned all my blankets, carpets, and work instruments out of jealousy. I survived. This was in 1939–1940. But the most difficult period of my life came later."

A Lineage of Married Yogins

"Later my guru wrote me that I should get married. I did not want to. Then Krishnamacharya told me that he belonged to a lineage of married yogins and that if I did not want to get married I could no longer call him my guru. But the choice of my wife was not made, according to tradition, by comparing our two horoscopes; and it was not Guruji who chose my wife. I saw a girl who came to the house with my sisters, and I decided to get married."

Advice of the Guru

"One day after doing pranayama, I was practicing Corpse Pose (relaxation) and lost consciousness. But inside I was full of awareness, as if in the middle of a sea: full of peace, lightness and light. I immediately wrote Krishnamacharya to find out what to do. He answered that it was a very good experience, but that I definitely should not try to make it happen again. Kundalini awakens when it wants to and how it wants to. We are not on earth to enjoy life. If such moments present themselves, enjoy them fully, but don't look for them. If you do, you leave the straight path and cut yourself off from any possibility of further evolution. The past is the past. You must live in the present.

"I practiced yoga almost despite myself; I did not feel like it but felt obliged to return to the mat. Then one night I had a dream: Lord Venkateswara, the God who protects our family, appeared to me and smiled. With one hand, he blessed me, and with the other, he gave me a grain of rice. The next morning, I wrote Guruji to ask him an explanation of this dream. He answered that from now on God would feed us and take care of us, that I no longer needed to be concerned about it, and that we would no longer be short of anything. That gave me great joy, because at that time life was still very hard.

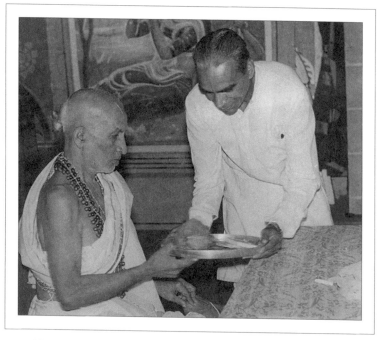

IYENGAR PRESENTS AN OFFERING TO KRISHNAMACHARYA, PUNE, 1961

From that moment on, it was no longer the yoga that stuck to me, it was me who stuck to yoga. And as you see, we are very poor but lack for nothing; the children are well fed and behave."

Veneration

Krishnamacharya is to Iyengar the venerated and respected guru. One day he told me, "My guru is a lot better than I am in pranayama, but to devote himself more deeply to the practice of pranayama he has abandoned the practice of asana. In asana I am better than he is. Right now, between the two of us, we encompass the wholeness of yoga," he laughed. This was in 1960. Since then, who can tell how far the countless hours of daily practice have taken him?

One day, after a lot of urging, Krishnamacharya agreed to come up to Pune. That created a lot of emotion in the family. The following is a letter dated November 13, 1961, that relates the event:

"We had Guruji here during ten days. At my request, he passed by on his way to Varanasi. He gave several conferences where he took Geeta and Vanita (the two oldest girls) to demonstrate the poses. Many people came to visit us to see him. We all were on our feet from four in the morning till ten at night, without a break. He was impressed with my work and with the interest I had generated here and in Bombay. After twenty-two years of persistent requests, he has come to my home. He told me that he was proud of me and blessed us all."

Gratitude

On his way back, Krishnamacharya stopped in again. In this letter of November 29, you can feel the emotion, joy, and devotion of Iyengar:

"My venerated teacher has come again and has blessed me intensely. His blessing will make deep inroads in me. He observed me while I was teaching, and when I practiced asana and pranayama he was impressed. He also organized a special public ceremony with the help of my students and presented me with a gold medal. He awarded me with a title he had engraved on the medal: Yoganga Shikshaka Chakravarti, which means 'King among the teachers of yoga.'

"He also had diplomas printed to award to the students. You will get yours by separate mail; it is signed by both of us, him and me.

"He did not teach me anything new; his blessing will really bring the true path and new approaches into view. I will send you pictures."

In another letter he again spoke of the celebration that was organized for him by the guru and was such a special event. This guru, once so severe, so remote, so impressive, suddenly recognized all the work that his severity and advice had triggered, and he approved. It was an unforgettable day.

The oldest son of Krishnamacharya, Shri Shrinivasan, was one of seven Brahmins that officiated at the inauguration of the Ramamani Iyengar Memorial Yoga Institute, in Pune, in January of 1975. A close relationship exists between Iyengar and Shri Shrinivasan.

The Artist

"Look at this pose," he said during a demonstration in Geneva. "Physically speaking it is perfect, technically speaking nothing is missing, but it is dead. There is no unity, because I am speaking to you at the same time. I have not created *wholeness*. Now look closely. I am going to unify everything in me, and then the pose will have life, will shine." And what passionate transformation we witnessed that afternoon! The artisan became an artist, the genius had left behind the technique of the craftsman, and he offered us a masterpiece. It was beautiful and touching. He did it again to be sure that everyone could see the difference, understand it, and incorporate it in their own life.

"Judgment or understanding on one hand, dexterity on the other, must work together in you. Adjust one by one. Each movement is an art. Using the word *art* without reaching this perfection has no meaning," he liked to explain. That day I understood that perfection of technique requires and provokes in the one who seeks it a progressive and constant refining of all mental and spiritual faculties. From soul to body and body to soul, the demand is transmitted to create the masterpiece that will be neither a beautiful physical pose nor a beautiful soul without a body, but an integration beyond duality.

Noëlle Is Also Rewarded

Iyengar knows how to inspire respect for the guru in his students, but he also knows how to reward their efforts with simple, well-chosen words.

After our time together in 1959, a session that brought me so much but cost a lot of pain and suffering, he dedicated a book to me with these kind words: "To my grateful and sincere painstaking Noëlle, etc." How well he had understood me, I was very happy!

When he came for the first time to supervise my work and give a class to my students in 1971, I felt ill at ease. We all did. He never gave me a compliment. He gave a dazzling session, and I awaited some verdict. He found an angle for letting me know his satisfaction without telling me directly: "Give me some paper, your dear mother must worry and I will put her at ease." And he wrote her a marvelous letter, the best certificate a sincere student could receive from an admired teacher:

"Noëlle's students did very good yoga. I am delighted to tell you that they all do well. Only master touch is required. Then the yoga in them blossoms. Her work is really good. May God bless her and you for having a disciplined daughter. She is an asset to you and to the Parisians who are interested in yoga. B.K.S. Iyengar, 26-6-71"

Afterword

Every position the people took delighted me; it was a joy to watch them move. They had an earthy, permanent quality, as if rooted to the soil. . . . I wanted to capture their timelessness. As they hovered near a fire, or bent over a whale, or cut a seal, they had natural grace of movement, without self-consciousness.

—Claire Fejes, *People of the Noatak*

IN 1959, IYENGAR gave Noëlle a clue that eventually transformed her teaching and understanding of yoga. "Walk behind Indian women," he said, "and observe them closely, copy them. When your shadow matches theirs, you will have made progress." Thus the idea of learning from people still living in balance, which Noëlle calls Aplomb, was present from the very beginning of her studies with Iyengar.

Another time that year, when she was working on standing postures, Noëlle suddenly felt Iyengar slide his foot under her front foot, causing her weight to shift to her heels. The pose instantly became light. This was Iyengar's way of teaching her about natural balance without using words, but she understood his intention only much later and after a lot of searching. For many years, the quality of lightness that comes from a balanced pose remained elusive.

In Paris, during a seminar with Iyengar in 1971, the students were in Shoulderstand (Sarvangasana). He said: "All the necks are hard. You are going to have problems. Let them come down." That whole year, Noëlle and her students explored how to make the neck relax, and they succeeded, but the posture was rounded. In 1972 Iyengar happened to pass through Paris again. Again the students were in Sarvangasana. The master shot daggers at Noëlle: "They are not on the axis, that's clear!" The message then was that the neck should be relaxed and the pose vertical, *on the axis*, to enable extension. Noëlle says, "For the first time, the word *axis* hit me."

In the crucial year of 1976, Iyengar returned to teach in Paris, and within three days Noëlle had several major revelations. First, at the exhibition of Ancient Egyptian art at the Grand Palais, Iyengar said something surprising about the statue of Ramses: "All this Western art falls forward. You would think that the sculptor wants to bring our attention to the feet." Then at the Guimet Museum of Asian Art, before the great Rajanaga made of pink sandstone, he exclaimed: "Look, with us that rises."

During a memorable class, Iyengar demonstrated how sitting on the floor in Baddha Konasana (Tailor Pose), he could not keep his back straight. He explained that when the weight of the pelvis falls backwards, all the back muscles must make a huge effort to keep the back straight. The play of weight and counterweight relative to the axis of the body is not respected, and this interferes with breathing, as well.

Next, he sat perched on a pile of blankets, explaining that the weight of the pelvis must fall forward to be in balance and respect the natural arch at the lower lumbar spine. To do this, the knees—being slender—should be a little lower than the upper thigh. In this position, the femur is horizontal. Thus he recommended that Westerners no longer sit directly on the floor but use supports adapted individually.

On the last of these three fantastic days, Iyengar taught what Noëlle now regards as the first class of Aplomb (Balance). Taking as his theme the comma, question mark, and exclamation point, he illustrated the three positions with three men placed in front of the group. The student with a rounded back he called "comma"; the one standing straight and leaning back he called "question mark." The third was a country boy who had never done yoga in his life but stood comfortably planted on both feet, straight and open. Iyengar made him the good example and called him "exclamation point."

By the spring of 1981, Noëlle's approach to the postures had changed radically. Everything became lighter. What appeared insignificant had become fundamental. She had a kind of spiritual catharsis and wrote some twenty books about everything yoga had taught her till then.

Next she began to sound the alarm about the dangers of a yoga that is transposed onto our Western constitutions without discretion. She tried to isolate the basic needs of a pose for an unbalanced Western body to replace the image of the pose executed on the axis by an Easterner who is used to sitting on the floor, has a different diet, and lives in a different climate. She developed ways to prevent injury while doing yoga.

Headstand (Sirsasana) especially posed a problem. As Noëlle relates: "When I would come down from Sirsasana I felt like there was a spider web over my face and my neck hurt, despite Iyengar's detailed instructions. So I thought that if I could find a woman who carries the equivalent of her own weight on her head, it might reveal some details that I had not yet understood."

She went to Africa, then to Portugal, to find people who were used to carrying loads on their heads. She even got permission to X-ray their spines and collected about a hundred tests. She found that nobody carries as much as their own weight. People learn to carry progressively heavier loads, and extension of the entire spine is essential.

A key discovery emerged from the X-rays: everyone who carries on the head has a very pronounced lower lumbar arch and the major joints are aligned for proper balance. This way, most of the weight is transferred to the heels "to a surface the size of a coin" (Iyengar, 1959). Noëlle realized that nowadays few Westerners live in this kind of equilibrium. The knowledge of "being in balance" seemed to be lost. She had to help people to rediscover it.

To carry out her new mission, Noëlle created the Institut Supérieur d'Aplomb, located next to the already existing Institut de Yoga B.K.S. Iyengar. Its mission has been to teach the public how to maintain health and vitality.

Noëlle considers Aplomb as pure yoga, a continuation of her work with Iyengar, in which the most natural poses of everyday life are themselves asana. The teacher tries to open the eyes and awaken the senses of the student. The student digests, not by memorizing postures and directions, but by discovering the law of balance, the mysteries of the human skeleton, the trap of tension, and the capacity to go always further into relaxation. To practice with attention in every moment is to be on a road to perfection as taught by Iyengar.

Georgia and Philippe Leconte

Glossary

abhyasa: constant and determined practice

ahimsa: nonharming; nonviolence

ananda: bliss; spiritual joy

Ardhanarisvara: a deity depicted as half male and half female, the right half representing the Lord Siva and the left half, his consort Parvati

artha: purpose

asana: posture

Atman, Atma: the Soul; the Self

Atma-darsan: experience of the Self; enlightenment; Self-realization

bhakti: devotion; love; adoration; worship

Brahma: the Supreme Being; the Creator; the first deity of Hindu trinity

brahmacarya: a life of celibacy, religious study, and self-restraint

buddhi: discrimination; wisdom

chakra: plexus; wheel

chela: pupil

citta: the mind in its total or collective sense, composed of three categories: mind, reason, and ego

darsan: vision; sight

dharana: concentration

dharma: moral or religious prescription; virtue

dhoti: a cloth worn by men around the waist

dhyana: meditation

ekagrata: one-pointedness; fixed on one object or point only

guru: teacher; mentor; one who leads from darkness into light

hatha: force; will

Hatha Yoga: the yoga of will and discipline whose goal is union with the Supreme

Hatha Yoga Pradipika: oldest surviving text on Hatha Yoga, dating from the fifteenth century

japa: repetitive prayer

jivatma: the individual or personal soul

jnana: wisdom; sacred knowledge derived from meditation on the higher truths of religion and philosophy

jnana-atman: self-knowledge

karma: action

kumbha: water pot; pitcher

kumbhaka: retention of the breath

kundalini: female serpent; divine cosmic energy; serpent power

lalata: forehead

linga: a stylized phallus worshipped as a symbol of the god Siva

mantra: a sacred thought or prayer; sacred syllables

moksa: liberation

mudra: a seal; a sealing posture; symbolic gesture

niyama: self-purification by discipline; the second of the eight limbs of yoga

om: the creating sound

Paramatma: Supreme Spirit; Universal Soul

Patanjali: the propounder of yoga philosophy

prakriti: nature

pramana: cognition; perception

prana: breath; respiration; life; vitality; energy

pranayama: rhythmic control of the breath

prasanta: peace and balance

pratyahara: withdrawal of the senses

puraka: inhalation of the breath

Purusa: the universal cosmic male from whose body the world was created

raja: king

recaka: exhalation of the breath

rishi: inspired sage

sadhak: seeker

sadhana: practice; spiritual quest

sakti: power; energy

samadhi: ecstasy; meditative absorption; a state in which the aspirant is one with the object of his meditation, the Supreme Spirit

sannyasin: renunciant

satya: truth

siddhi: accomplishment; magical power

sloka: stanza

susumna: central channel

sutra: thread; aphorism

tantra: name of a religious doctrine

tapas: self-discipline; austerity

vidya: knowledge

yamas: moral and ethical disciplines; the first of the eight limbs of yoga

yoga-darsana: the philosophy of yoga as propounded by Patanjali

yogasala: yoga studio

yogin: male yoga practitioner

Permissions

GRATEFUL ACKNOWLEDGMENT is made to Noëlle Perez-Christiaens for permission to translate and adapt her material for this book:

"Noëlle's India Journal": Adapted from *Un Mystique Hindou Ivre de Dieu: B.K.S. Iyengar* by Noëlle Perez-Christiaens (Paris: Institut de Yoga B.K.S. Iyengar, copyright © 1976).

"Sparks of Divinity": From *Etincelles de Divinité (Sparks of Divinity)*, compiled by Noëlle Perez-Christiaens (Paris: Institut de Yoga B.K.S. Iyengar, copyright © 1976).

"The Early Life of B.K.S. Iyengar": Adapted from *Un Mystique Hindou Ivre de Dieu: B.K.S. Iyengar* by Noëlle Perez-Christiaens (Paris: Institut de Yoga B.K.S. Iyengar, copyright © 1976).

We thank Steve Baczewski, for giving us permission to use his striking photograph of B. K. S. Iyengar on the cover. (This photograph originally appeared on the cover of *Yoga Journal*, July/August 1976.)

About the Authors

BORN IN 1925, Noëlle Perez-Christiaens was one of the first Westerners to study with B.K.S. Iyengar in Pune. Inspired by Iyengar's teaching, she searched for the principles of natural balance by observing the posture and movement of indigenous people around the world, and began to share her discoveries under the name of Aplomb as a basis for the practice of yoga as well as for everyday life. Altogether she has published twenty-seven books on yoga and Aplomb. In 2008, Noëlle received the degree of Doctor of Ethnophysiology from the Ecole des Hautes Etudes en Sciences Sociales in Paris for her work on Aplomb.

BORN IN 1945, Georgia Leconte began studying with Noëlle Perez-Christiaens in 1968. Today she is one of her closest collaborators, having devoted her life to yoga and Aplomb. In 1975, Georgia married Philippe Leconte, a physicist. Both of them have studied yoga with B.K.S. Iyengar. In 1976, they translated his classic work, *Light on Yoga*, into French. Georgia and Philippe also helped edit the original version of *Sparks of Divinity*.

From the Publisher

Rodmell Press publishes books on yoga, Buddhism, aikido, and Taoism. In the Bhagavadgita it is written, "Yoga is skill in action." It is our hope that our books will help individuals develop a more skillful practice—one that brings peace to their daily lives and to the earth. We thank all those whose support, encouragement, and practical advice sustain us in our efforts.

Catalog Request
(510) 841-3123 or (800) 841-3123
(510) 841-3123 (fax)
info@rodmellpress.com
www.rodmellpress.com

Trade Sales/United States, International
Publishers Group West
(800) 788-3123
(510) 528-5511 (sales fax)
info@pgw.com
www.pgw.com

Foreign Language and Book Club Rights
Linda Cogozzo, Publisher
(510) 841-3123
linda@rodmellpress.com
www.rodmellpress.com

Index

A

abhyasa (practice), 132. *See also* sadhana
   (practice, work, spiritual quest)
action
   analysis in, 109, 182, 185
   challenge and response in, 182, 186
   circumferential, 159
   dedicating to the Lord, 159
   disciplining mind through, 97, 138
   doing completely, 106
   doing one's best, 117
   doing versus not doing, 83
   dull versus intelligent, 185
   harmony in, 183
   humility in, 183
   knowing the source of, 188
   meditation in, 171
   movement versus, 187–188, 189
   oneness in, 47
   passivity in, 185
   Patanjali on intelligence and, 135
   personality mirrored by, 159
   to please another, 81
   poise in, 117
   precision in, 118
   psychological, converting yoga into, 136
   reflecting on, 189
   relaxation after, 186
   relaxation in, 137, 163
   right, propaganda contained by, 183
   by Self, not intelligence, 176
   sensory, 183
   silence with, 102
   with soul, 165
   space between silence and, 159
   stopping overactivity, 92
   tension versus, 142
   translating physical into spiritual, 134
   without thinking, 107
   words without, 139
   work required for, 181
   in yoga, 64
age of determination, 110
aging, 132, 157
ahimsa (nonviolence or nonharming)
   anger in classes and, 129–130
   described, 43
   nonviolent yoga, 191
   translation of, 69
analysis in action, 109, 182, 185
ananda (bliss, joy)
   in failure and success, 67
   in Savasana, 104
   as unity, 41
   as worth all effort, 39

receptive, 151
eating with fingers, 30–31
education, meaning of, 113
ego, using as an instrument, 170
egoists, 131
Elizabeth, queen of Belgium
  conversation with Iyengar, 52
  lessons given to, 202
  photographs with Iyengar, 53, 106
emotions
  control needed for meditation, 97
  developing for divine purposes, 159
  immaturity of Westerners, 85, 93
energy. *See also* kundalini
  letting flow from feet, 136
  merging intelligence with flow of, 190
  moving with the flow of, 163
enquiry, 176, 188
escapism, 188
eternity, 174
ethics and morality
  asana and, 168
  beginning in us, 87
  ethical diet, 121
  ethical framework, 40
  immoral yoga, 179
  religion and, 129
  of teaching, 188
exclamation mark posture, 217
excuses, ignoring, 40, 83
exhalation. *See also* inhalation; pranayama
  as art of surrender, 155
  awareness and, 152
  flowing inside, 169
  with movement, 187
  path of expiration, 166
  soul into Universal Consciousness, 166
  surrender to God during, 17, 37
  toward the heart, 104
  without tension, 152–153
extension
  freedom brought by, 130, 160

of the mind, 178
  relaxation following, 184
  relaxation in, 189
  synchronizing horizontal and vertical, 175
external, converting to internal, 187
extroversion, 134, 188
eye, single, 142, 166
eyes
  all over the body, 178, 189
  in asana, 65, 122
  closing, 151
  Iyengar's millions of, 192
  keeping open for awareness, 145–146
  observation from mind, not eyes, 103
  open, consciousness symbolized by,
    24–25
  opening wide, 169
  in relaxation, 161
  in skin, 119, 138
  understanding and, 166

F
faith, poise in action and, 117
fatigue, teaching and, 82
fear
  guru's help for chela's, 99
  importance of mastering, 63
feeling
  as the eye, 166
  observation and, 138
feet, letting energy flow from, 136
Fejes, Claire, 215
financial security
  challenges of, 95
  Gita on, 96
  need for, 57
fingers, eating with, 30–31
forgiveness, justice and, 181
freedom
  bearing pain required for, 173
  in the body, 46
  in body, before spiritual light, 164

hate, 160
Hatha Yoga, 113, 127, 171
Hatha Yoga Pradipika, 16, 20, 28, 35
head and neck balance, 99
head balance, 174, 183
Headstand (Sirsasana), 143, 218
health
  body forgotten in, 88
  building, 46
  as harmony, 49
  Iyengar's care for Noëlle's, 10–11
  mind affected by, 87
  in modern world, yoga and, 110
  needed for finding truth, 46
  as perfect balance, 112, 113
  sound mind in sound body, 51
  yoga as only means of keeping, 161
Homji, Mrs., 6
human nature, pruning, 178
humility or humbleness
  in action, 183
  as art of learning, 161, 193
  beginning of, 163
  inside, strength outside, 193
  in intellect, 91
  in meditation, 153
  needed in sadhana, 190
  teaching, 193

I

ideas as obstacles, 167, 186
impersonality cult, 155
impotency, 161, 189
India
  spiritual gifts of, 84
  touch in, 198
  Western intelligence versus Indian, 146–147
  yoga as international, not Indian, 125
infinite, going to, 145
inhalation. *See also* exhalation; pranayama
  like clouds spreading in the sky, 103

  path on inspiration, 166
  receiving life from God during, 17, 37
  without disturbing consciousness, 121
injury
  not being deterred by, 59
  treatment of Noëlle's sprained back, 22–24
inquisitive spirit, need for, 99
Institut Supérieur d'Aplomb, 218
intellect
  accurate or defective asana and, 184
  developing for divine purposes, 159
  of head and heart, 89, 90
  humility needed in, 91
  meditation as adjustment of, 171
  meditative, 138
  mobility of, 182
  sensitivity and, 180
  stable, 182
intelligence
  analytical versus practical, 93
  for balance, strength versus, 108
  body, 84, 158, 178
  of brain versus heart, 182
  in contact with movement, 164
  descending versus ascending, 183
  developing, 148
  dull versus intelligent action, 185
  even, like a full river, 133
  everywhere, 135, 142
  of the heart in meditation, 149
  Indian versus Western, 146–147
  intoxicated, Self blocked by, 176
  maturity needed with, 190
  merging with the energy flow, 190
  needed for asana, 75
  Patanjali on action and, 135
  physical versus mental, 162
  projecting from the source, 130
  sincerity paired with, 183
  too much of, 142
  uninterrupted, 167

light
  dependent on pain, 131
  inner and outer, 165
listening, by introverts, 182
liver trouble, 187
Lord. *See* God
lotus metaphor, 49
Lotus Pose, 50
Loustic (Noëlle's mother's dog), 108
love
  for the body, 137
  described, 47
  honesty in, 133
  human needed to know Divine, 174
  incarnating, 65
  of Iyengar for pupils, 142
  language of, 174
  meditation as acting with, 77
  as merciless, 170
  pupils,' blessing of, 57
  in yoga, 64
low blood pressure, 86

M
macrocosm, conquering, 177
Malcuzynski, W. (pianist), 98
manas chakra, 188
Mandalasana, 53
mantra, movement as, 172
Manusmriti, 69
marriage
  defined, 148
  of Iyengar and Ramamani, 11, 149,
    201–203, 210
maximum
  aiming at, 169–170
  expected of pupils, 111
  going beyond, 160, 162, 179–180
means versus end, 85
median line, watching, 99
medicine replaced by asana, 183
meditation

abstract, 171
as acting with love, 77
in action, 171
as adjustment of intellect, 171
artificial, 170
in asana, 7–8, 41
asana for, 105, 107
as being in a primitive state, 146
brain in, 137, 153, 165, 170, 172
breathing in, 152–153, 154
commonness found in, 171
concentration versus, 133, 170
concrete and abstract, 152–153
concrete to abstract, 96, 105
as deep sleep in wakeful state, 142
dhyana, defined, 44
emotional control needed for, 97
falling upon you, 61
heart drawn to Lord in, 90
as highest form of surrender, 170
humility in, 153
intelligence of the heart in, 149
looking with ears in, 119
mind sharpened by, 90
no movement in brain and mind in, 154
as oneness, 61, 141
pins and needles during, 174
posture as, 140
pranayama as, 17, 37, 84
silence in silence as beginning of, 76
space between skull and brain for, 170
stability needed in, 169
still brain needed for, 172
as timeless, 73
tranquility of senses versus, 150
transcendental, 126
universal consciousness in, 149
yoga as, 138
meditative intellect, 138
memory, usefulness of, 85, 145
Menuhin, Yehudi
  Iyengar invited to Europe by, 3, 197

Rajanaga statue, 216
rajas, 176
Ramananda, Swami, 199
Ramses statue, 216
reincarnation, 113–114
relaxation
  in action, 137, 163
  action followed by, 186
  of body and brain, 135
  coming to yoga for, 164
  complete, 39
  as emptiness, 65
  in extension, 189
  extension followed by, 184
  mastering the art of, 96
  relaxing pupils before strenuous
    poses, 191
  skin and eyes in, 161
  in sleep, 38
  stillness in, 166
  stretching and, 162
  stretching completely as, 138
  trying versus doing, 192
religion
  degeneration of, 15
  as knowing thyself, 168
  morality and, 129
  yoga as culture rather than, 188
  yoga as science of, 191
  yoga's affect on, 135
religiousness
  irreligious work, 165
  nature of, 92
  religious mind, 86
  within, 168
retention (kumbhaka). *See also*
    pranayama
  breath holding you in, 150
  conscious versus unconscious, 16–17
  as God entering the body, 143
  silence with, 121
  state of suspense in, 155

  at top of chest, 122
ribs, as wings of the body, 122
Rodmell Press, 224
root, correcting from, 95

S

sadhaka, 132
sadhana (practice, work, spiritual quest)
  as abhyasa, 132
  determination in, 42
  devoting to God, 58
  discipline of, 121
  doing more than you can, 40, 63
  ease with persistence in, 64
  effort needed in, 160
  hard, required for results, 36
  hardest road as shortest road, 190
  humility needed in, 190
  importance of, 57, 76
  irreligious, 165
  Iyengar's practice, 12–13, 20
  Noëlle's practice, 19
  not leaving for tomorrow, 35
  for others, 21
  as passion, 25
  Patanjali on, 12–13
  problems interfering with, 66
  pursuing sadhana at all cost, 64
  sharing, 39
  success due only to, 184
  uninterrupted, 141
  weaknesses dissolved by, 143
  wisdom through, 71
Sakti, in Trikonasana, 77
samadhi
  described, 44
  Raja Yoga as, 20
  as Self free from contact of things, 41
  as stillness with complete conscious-
    ness, 133
  strong nervous system needed for, 55
  swoon versus, 171

Upanishads
  stories from, 25, 70
  on training the body, 132
Uttanasana, 62

V

vanity or pride, 121, 141, 193
Venkateswara, Iyengar's dream of, 210
Vibhatijoti Swami, 199
vidya (acquired knowledge), 133. *See also*
  knowledge
violence in postures
  to balance, 174
  in the beginning, 95
  tight brain and, 191
  visible in face and practice, 108
Virabhadrasana I, 48
Virabhadrasana III, 66
Virasana, 105
virility, 161, 189
void, 13
Voyage d'une Parisienne à Lhassa (Neel), 2

W

walking, technique for, 121
weaknesses, spiritual advancement versus,
  105
wealth
  as within, 108
  financial security, 57, 95, 96
Westerners
  emotional immaturity of, 85, 93
  objective intelligence of, 146–147
will of God, surrender to
  about the shape things take, 65
  in exceeding one's capacity, 64
  in regard to earnings, 50, 57, 59
  in regard to rebirth, 91
will or will power
  discipline developing, 35
  "hatha" meaning will, 130
  intellect needed for, 168

practice developing, 42
strong buttocks for, 38
will over will, 168
wings of the body, ribs as, 122
wisdom (buddhi)
  discrimination versus, 84
  as earned, 182
  through work, 71
  through yoga, 120
  vidya versus, 133
work. *See* sadhana

Y

yama, 43
yawning, stopping, 186
yoga. *See also* asana (poses or postures);
    spiritual and physical yoga
  alert and agile mind from, 111
  ancient requirements for, 92
  as an art, 86, 112, 128, 130
  artificial divisions of, 127
  in asana, 160
  as balancing sides of the body, 76
  as beauty in observation, 167
  benefits of, 100, 165
  body as beginning of, 100
  body, not brain, as instructor for, 185
  books on, 13, 16
  character built by, 120, 128
  as circulation, 36
  complete awareness as aim of, 92
  as concentration, 71
  concentration not needed for, 148
  as controlling the mind, 73
  converting to psychological action, 136
  correspondence course in, 173
  as culture, not religion, 188
  doing in society, 157
  eight steps in asana, 164
  eight steps of, 38
  for everyone, 157
  everything embraced by, 120